USMLE ROAD MAP

PHARMACOLOGY

BERTRAM KATZUNG, MD, PhD

Professor Emeritus
Department of Cellular and Molecular Pharmacology
University of California, San Francisco

ANTHONY TREVOR, PhD

Professor Emeritus
Department of Cellular and Molecular Pharmacology
University of California, San Francisco

Lange Medical Books/McGraw-Hill
Medical Publishing Division

New York   Chicago   San Francisco   Lisbon   London   Madrid   Mexico City
Milan   New Delhi   San Juan   Seoul   Singapore   Sydney   Toronto

The McGraw·Hill Companies

USMLE Road Map: Pharmacology, Second Edition

Copyright © 2006, 2003 by The McGraw-Hill Companies, Inc. All rights reserved. Printed in the United States of America. Except as permitted under the United States Copyright Act of 1976, no part of this publication may be reproduced or distributed in any form or by any means, or stored in a data base or retrieval system, without prior written permission of the publisher.

1234567890 DOC/DOC 098765

ISBN: 0-07-144581-1

ISSN: 1543-5814

Notice

Medicine is an ever-changing science. As new research and clinical experience broaden our knowledge, changes in treatment and drug therapy are required. The authors and the publisher of this work have checked with sources believed to be reliable in their efforts to provide information that is complete and generally in accord with the standards accepted at the time of publication. However, in view of the possibility of human error or changes in medical sciences, neither the authors nor the publisher nor any other party who has been involved in the preparation or publication of this work warrants that the information contained herein is in every respect accurate or complete, and they disclaim all responsibility for any errors or omissions or for the results obtained from use of the information contained in this work. Readers are encouraged to confirm the information contained herein with other sources. For example and in particular, readers are advised to check the product information sheet included in the package of each drug they plan to administer to be certain that the information contained in this work is accurate and that changes have not been made in the recommended dose or in the contraindications for administration. This recommendation is of particular importance in connection with new or infrequently used drugs.

This book was set in Adobe Garamond by Pine Tree Composition.
The editors were Jason Malley, Karen Edmonson, and Regina Y. Brown.
The production supervisor was Catherine H. Saggese.
The illustration manager was Charissa Baker.
Graphics and illustrations created by Dragonfly Media Group.
The index was prepared by Jerry Rayla.

RR Donnelley was printer and binder.

This book is printed on acid-free paper

CONTENTS

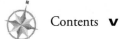

USING THE
USMLE ROAD MAP SERIES
FOR SUCCESSFUL REVIEW

What Is the Road Map Series?

Short of having your own personal tutor, the USMLE Road Map Series is the best source for efficient review of major concepts and information in the medical sciences.

Why Do You Need A Road Map?

It allows you to navigate quickly and easily through your pharmacology course notes and textbook and prepares you for USMLE and course examinations.

How Does the Road Map Series Work?

Outline Form: Connects the facts in a conceptual framework so that you understand the ideas and retain the information.

Color and Boldface: Highlights words and phrases that trigger quick retrieval of concepts and facts.

Clear Explanations: Are fine-tuned by years of student interaction. The material is written by authors selected for their excellence in teaching and their experience in preparing students for board examinations.

Illustrations: Provide the vivid impressions that facilitate comprehension and recall.

 Clinical Correlations: Link all topics to their clinical applications, promoting fuller understanding and memory retention.

 Clinical Problems: Give you valuable practice for the clinical vignette-based USMLE questions.

 Explanations of Answers: Are learning tools that allow you to pinpoint your strengths and weaknesses.

Acknowledgments

Our thanks to Jason Malley, Karen Edmonson, and Regina Y. Brown
for their editorial efforts.

CHAPTER 1
GENERAL PRINCIPLES OF PHARMACOLOGY

I. Definitions

A. **Pharmacology** is the science of the interaction of chemicals with living systems at the molecular level.

B. **Toxicology** is the area of pharmacology that deals with the undesirable effects of chemicals on living systems.

C. **Drugs** are chemicals that alter the function of living systems by interactions at the molecular level. These functional changes may be beneficial (therapeutic) or toxic.

D. **Drug-binding sites** are the components of living systems with which drugs interact. If the binding of a drug results in a functional change, the binding site is called a *receptor.* If no alteration in function results from drug binding, the binding site is called an *inert binding site.*

E. **Pharmacokinetics** describes the actions of biological systems on drugs, including absorption, distribution, and elimination.

F. **Pharmacodynamics** describes the detailed actions of drugs on living systems.

II. Pharmacokinetic Principles

A. Movement of Drugs in the Body

1. To be absorbed and distributed, drugs must cross barriers such as the intestinal wall and the blood–brain barrier. This requires passive diffusion or active transport.

2. **Passive diffusion** across lipid membranes requires some degree of lipid solubility.

   a. **Lipid solubility** is determined in part by the electrical charge on the molecule.

   b. For weak acids and weak bases (which comprise the majority of drugs), the charge is determined by the pH of the medium according to the **Henderson–Hasselbalch equation:**

$$\text{Log (protonated form/unprotonated form)} = pK_a - pH$$

   where the protonated form of a weak acid is the uncharged, more lipid-soluble form, and the unprotonated form of a weak base is the uncharged, more lipid-soluble form (Figure 1–1).

3. **Active transport** of drugs by special carrier molecules occurs if the drugs are structurally related to endogenous molecules such as amino acids or sugars.

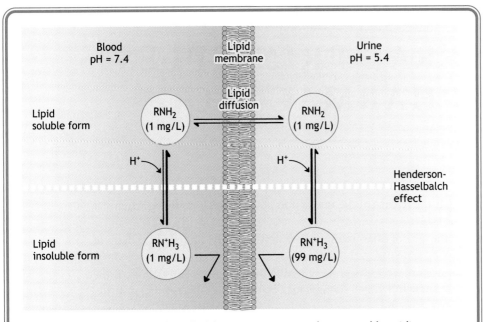

Figure 1–1. Henderson–Hasselbalch trapping occurs when a weakly acidic or weakly basic drug equilibrates across a membrane separating regions of different pH. For a weak base such as the hypothetical drug shown here (pK_a = 7.4), the region with lower pH (greater proton concentration) will trap more drug because the protonated form is less lipid soluble and cannot diffuse back across the membrane. The Henderson–Hasselbalch equation predicts that if the total concentration of this weak base in the blood at pH 7.4 is 2 mg/L (50% neutral, 50% protonated), the equilibrium concentration in the urine at pH 5.4 will be 100 mg/L (1 mg/L unprotonated, 99 mg/L protonated). This principle is used in detoxification of patients who have overdosed: excretion will be accelerated by acidifying the urine if the patient took a weak base, or alkalinizing if the patient took a weak acid.

Some very large or very polar drugs (vitamin B_{12}, iron) are complexed with proteins and actively transported into cells by endocytosis.

4. The **size of the drug molecule** also affects how readily a drug moves within the body.

   a. Very small molecules (lithium, alcohols, and gases) diffuse rapidly into most parts of the body.

   b. Large protein molecules (thrombolytic enzymes and botulinum toxin) diffuse very poorly.

B. Absorption

   1. Drugs may be administered directly at their site of action or they may be **absorbed** into the circulation to be distributed to distant sites of action.

   2. There are numerous **routes of administration.**

   a. **Intravenous** administration provides instantaneous and complete absorption.

b. The **oral** route is the most common route of administration because of its convenience, but for most drugs absorption is slower and less complete than with other routes.

c. Most other routes of administration (eg, **intramuscular, subcutaneous,** and **rectal**) fall between these two extremes.

d. The **transdermal** route, in which a drug is slowly released from a special vehicle, is used for prolonged action.

DRUG ABSORPTION

CLINICAL CORRELATION

Special formulations are often used to modify the rate of absorption of drugs. For example, intramuscular injection of drugs dissolved in oil provides for slow absorption; oral intake of drugs encapsulated in slowly-dissolving shells provides for similarly slow, continuous absorption.

3. **First-pass effect** refers to the elimination that occurs when a drug is first absorbed from the intestine and passes through the liver via the portal circulation. Because the liver is the primary drug-metabolizing organ of the body, drugs that are easily metabolized have a large first-pass effect and low bioavailability.

4. **Bioavailability** (*F*) for any given route of administration is calculated from a graph of plasma concentration versus time. The area under the plasma-concentration curve (AUC) is used to quantitate absorption into the systemic circulation:

$$F = AUC_{(route)}/AUC_{(IV)}$$

C. **Distribution**

1. Once absorbed into the bloodstream, drugs are distributed to other tissues.

2. The rate and extent of distribution depend on several factors.

a. **Blood flow to the tissue:** Tissues with high blood flow (viscera, brain, and muscle) will receive significant amounts of drug in a short time. Organs with low perfusion (fat and bone) will receive the drug more slowly.

b. **Size of the organ:** Very large organs (eg, skeletal muscle) can take up large quantities of drug if allowed to reach steady state.

c. **Solubility of the drug:** Drugs with high fat solubility will, at steady state, reach higher concentrations in tissues with high fat content (eg, adipose tissue and brain).

d. **Binding:** Drugs that bind to macromolecules in a tissue may be restricted in distribution. For example, drugs that bind avidly to plasma albumin (eg, warfarin) may be effectively restricted to the vascular compartment.

e. **Volume of distribution:** The volume of distribution (V_d) of a drug is a proportionality constant defined as

$$V_d = \text{amount of drug in the body/plasma concentration}$$

D. **Elimination**

1. Drugs are eliminated (their action is terminated) by metabolism to inactive molecular forms or by excretion. Metabolites of drugs must also eventually be excreted, but termination of action is of greater importance.

2. The vast majority of drugs follow **first-order elimination** kinetics, that is, rate of elimination is proportionate to plasma concentration (Figure 1–2A).

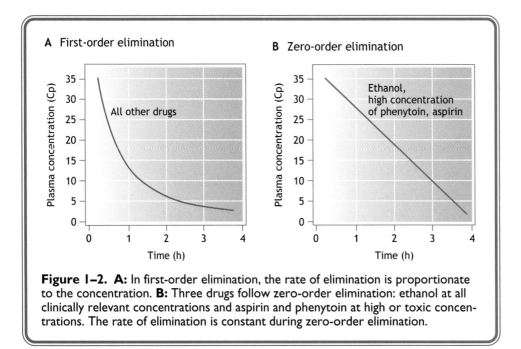

A First-order elimination

All other drugs

B Zero-order elimination

Ethanol, high concentration of phenytoin, aspirin

Figure 1–2. A: In first-order elimination, the rate of elimination is proportionate to the concentration. **B:** Three drugs follow zero-order elimination: ethanol at all clinically relevant concentrations and aspirin and phenytoin at high or toxic concentrations. The rate of elimination is constant during zero-order elimination.

    a. Only three clinically important drugs follow **zero-order** elimination kinetics (Figure 1–2B), that is, rate of elimination is fixed and independent of plasma concentration.

    b. Zero-order kinetics apply to ethanol at all clinically important concentrations and to phenytoin and aspirin at high concentrations.

  3. The elimination of drugs that follow first-order kinetics can be characterized by a proportionality constant, **clearance,** *Cl.* Clearance is defined as

$$Cl = \text{rate of elimination/plasma concentration}$$

  4. The elimination **half-life** ($t_{1/2}$) of drugs that follow first-order kinetics is defined as the time required (after distribution is complete) for the amount of drug in any compartment to fall by 50%. It can be derived from graphs of plasma concentration versus time (Figure 1–3), or it can be obtained by calculation:

$$t_{1/2} = 0.693 \times V_d / Cl$$

  5. For most drugs, elimination takes place by **hepatic metabolism** or **renal excretion.**

    a. A few drugs are also metabolized in the kidneys.

    b. Excretion of parent drugs and of drug metabolites is usually into the urine, but some drugs are excreted into the bile.

    c. Gases are usually excreted by way of the lungs.

  6. Drug metabolism involves two major chemical pathways.

    a. Phase I pathways involve alterations that make the drug more reactive and capable of combining with polar conjugating groups.

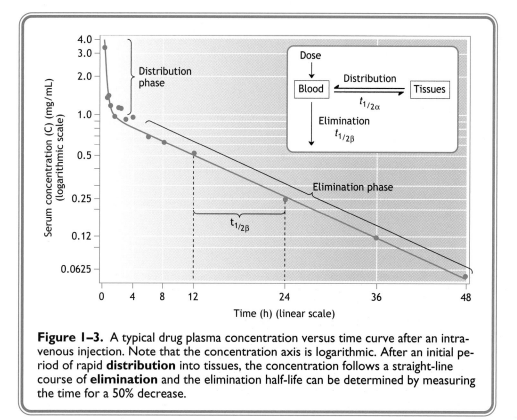

Figure 1–3. A typical drug plasma concentration versus time curve after an intravenous injection. Note that the concentration axis is logarithmic. After an initial period of rapid **distribution** into tissues, the concentration follows a straight-line course of **elimination** and the elimination half-life can be determined by measuring the time for a 50% decrease.

    b. Phase II pathways involve conjugation of a polar group (sulfate, acetate, and glucuronate) to the drug molecule.

  7. Phase I metabolism usually involves one or more members of a large family of hepatic enzymes called **cytochrome P-450** (**CYP450**) enzymes. The cytochrome enzymes catalyze oxidation (most important), reduction, and hydrolysis.

  8. The most important members of this CYP450 family (1A2, 2C9, 2D6, and 3A4) and others are susceptible to **inhibition** by certain drugs, and **amplification (induction)** by others. Such inhibition or induction can result in important **drug–drug interactions.**

E. Dosage Regimens

  1. Calculation of a dosage regimen requires knowledge of the target therapeutic plasma concentration and the pharmacokinetic parameters for the drug in the patient.

  2. The **loading dose** must "fill" the volume of distribution of the drug (V_d) to achieve the target plasma concentration (C_p):

$$\text{Loading dose} = \frac{V_d \times C_p}{F}$$

3. The **maintenance dosage** must replace the drug that is being eliminated by the body over time to maintain a steady target plasma concentration (C_p), and thus involves clearance (Cl):

$$\text{Maintenance dosage} = \frac{Cl \times C_p}{F}$$

   a. The dosing interval for a maintenance dosing regimen is usually based on the drug's half-life such that peak and trough concentrations do not vary excessively from the target C_p.
   b. Most oral drugs are given one or more times a day but rarely more than four times a day.
   c. Drugs with very short half-lives may have to be given by a different route (eg, intravenous infusion) or in the form of slow- or extended-release oral formulations.

CORRECTION OF DOSAGE REGIMENS

CLINICAL CORRELATION

- **Correction of dosage regimens** may be necessary in a specific patient to account for variations in pharmacokinetics.
- The clearance of drugs may be significantly affected by disease. For instance, patients with severe hepatic or renal disease may have reduced clearance of drugs that are eliminated by these routes.
- In contrast, the volume of distribution is rarely changed significantly by disease.

III. Pharmacodynamic Principles

   A. **Receptor Types**
      1. Drug receptors can be divided into five groups.
      2. These groups have different locations and effects (Table 1–1).

   B. **Drug–Receptor Interactions**
      1. Most agonist (receptor-activating) and antagonist (receptor-blocking) drugs bind to their receptors with weak, reversible bonds.
      2. A few antagonists bind with strong, covalent bonds, resulting in irreversible action.

   C. **Graded Dose–Response Relationships**
      1. When an agonist drug is applied in increasing doses to a responsive system and the increments in activity are recorded, a graded dose–response curve is obtained (Figure 1–4). Binding of the drug to its receptors follows a similar curve.
      2. Two important properties of the drug can be derived from this plot: the **concentration or dose for half-maximal effect** ($\mathbf{EC_{50}}$ or $\mathbf{ED_{50}}$) and the **maximum effect** ($\mathbf{E_{max}}$).
         a. The EC_{50} is a measure of the potency of the drug and its affinity for its receptor.
         b. The E_{max} is a measure of the maximum response that can be expected from the drug in this system.
         c. The corresponding measures for concentration-binding plots are $\mathbf{K_d}$ and $\mathbf{B_{max}}$.

   D. **Quantal Dose–Response Relationships**
      1. When a specific intensity of drug response is defined and the doses required to produce that intensity of response are measured in a large population of sub-

Table 1–1. Types of drug receptors.

Receptor Type	Action	Location	Drug Examples
Steroid	Modulates gene expression in the cell nucleus	Cytoplasm or nucleus	Estrogen, corticosteroid, thyroid hormone
Ion channel	Opens to permit ion diffusion	Cell membrane	Acetylcholine (on nicotinic acetylcholine receptor)
Transmembrane tyrosine kinase	Phosphorylates cytoplasmic proteins	Cell membrane	Insulin
JAK-STAT	Activates a cytoplasmic protein kinase (STAT)	Cell membrane and cytoplasm	Cytokines
G protein-coupled	Activates a membrane G protein that modulates an enzyme or channel	Cell membrane	Norepinephrine, acetylcholine (on muscarinic receptor)

jects, biologic variation results in a spread of these doses over a range (Figure 1–5).

2. The defined response may be a therapeutic or a toxic effect. Comparison of the median dose to produce a toxic effect versus the median dose to produce a therapeutic effect may be carried out to determine a **therapeutic index** (**TI**).

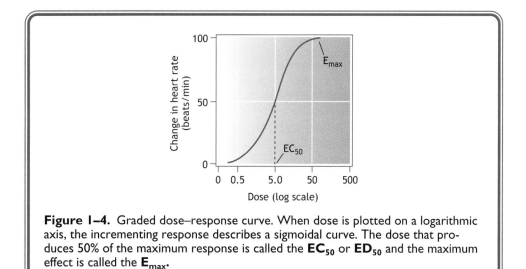

Figure 1–4. Graded dose–response curve. When dose is plotted on a logarithmic axis, the incrementing response describes a sigmoidal curve. The dose that produces 50% of the maximum response is called the **EC_{50}** or **ED_{50}** and the maximum effect is called the **E_{max}**.

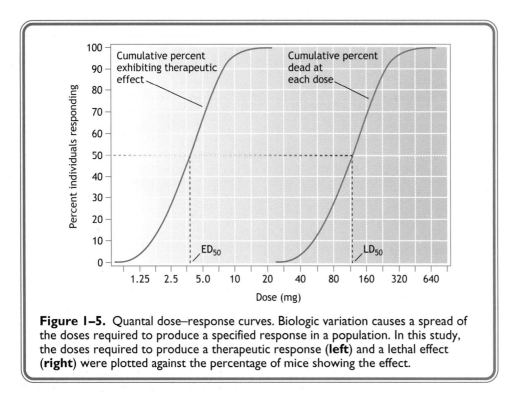

Figure I–5. Quantal dose–response curves. Biologic variation causes a spread of the doses required to produce a specified response in a population. In this study, the doses required to produce a therapeutic response (**left**) and a lethal effect (**right**) were plotted against the percentage of mice showing the effect.

$$TI = TD_{50}/ED_{50}$$

3. The therapeutic index is sometimes used in research to compare the safety of different members of a family of drugs.

E. Drug–Drug Antagonism

1. A drug that binds to a drug receptor site without activating it acts as an antagonist.

2. Similarly, a drug that binds to any portion of a receptor molecule and inactivates it through a chemical action will antagonize the action of agonists.

3. **Competitive pharmacologic antagonism:** Reversible binding to the receptor site that can be surmounted by an agonist will increase the measured EC_{50} of the agonist drug but have no effect on the E_{max} (Figure 1–6A).

4. **Irreversible pharmacologic antagonism:** Irreversible binding that cannot be surmounted at any concentration of agonist will decrease the E_{max}, but will not affect the EC_{50} for agonists (Figure 1–6B). However, if spare receptors are present, the EC_{50} will be shifted to the right by low doses of the antagonist until all the spare receptors are blocked. Further increases in the antagonist dose will then decrease the E_{max}.

5. **Physiologic antagonism:** Binding of an agonist drug to a receptor that produces effects opposite to the effects of another agonist drug acting at a second receptor is called **physiologic antagonism.** Effects on E_{max} and EC_{50} are dose- and drug-dependent.

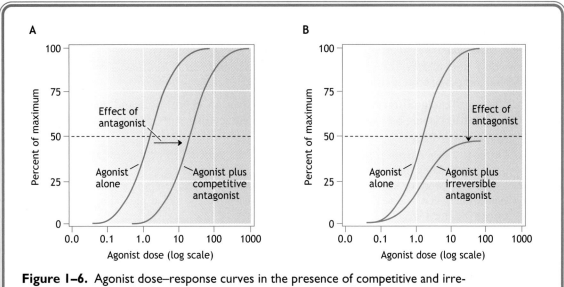

Figure 1–6. Agonist dose–response curves in the presence of competitive and irreversible antagonists. **A:** A competitive antagonist shifts the graded dose–response curve to the right but does not alter the maximum effect. **B:** An irreversible antagonist reduces the maximum effect but does not alter the ED_{50} unless spare receptors are present.

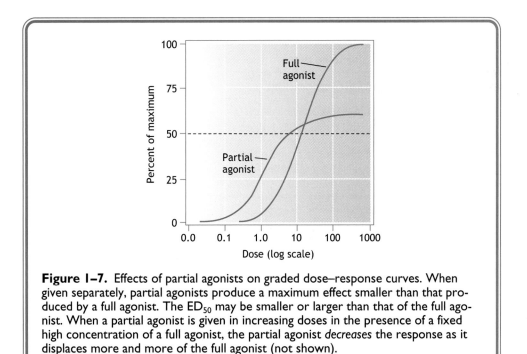

Figure 1–7. Effects of partial agonists on graded dose–response curves. When given separately, partial agonists produce a maximum effect smaller than that produced by a full agonist. The ED_{50} may be smaller or larger than that of the full agonist. When a partial agonist is given in increasing doses in the presence of a fixed high concentration of a full agonist, the partial agonist *decreases* the response as it displaces more and more of the full agonist (not shown).

PHYSIOLOGIC ANTAGONISTS

- *Physiologic antagonists* may be very effective and rapid acting.
- For example, epinephrine is the treatment of choice in anaphylaxis.
- In this potentially fatal condition epinephrine acts as a physiologic antagonist to leukotrienes and other mediators that do not act at epinephrine receptors.

  6. **Chemical antagonism:** A drug that chemically binds an agonist drug and prevents it from acting on its receptors is a chemical antagonist.

F. Partial Agonist Effect
  1. Drugs within a chemical family may all bind to the same receptor but not all produce the same maximum effect (E_{max}).
  2. Drugs that produce less than the full effect observed for that receptor system, even when given in doses that fully saturate the receptors, are called **partial agonists** (Figure 1–7).

Table 1–2. Types of drug tests.

Type of Test	Purpose	Subjects
Animal testing		
Pharmacological profile	Determine all useful or toxic actions of the drug and their mechanisms	Mice, rats, dogs, other
Reproductive toxicity	Detect fertility, teratogenic, and mutagenic effects	Mice, rats, rabbits, other
Chronic toxicity	Long-term testing for toxic effects	Mice, rats, other
Human trials (requires approval of an IND[1] application)		
Phase I	Determine the useful dose range, pharmacokinetics, and minimal toxic effects	25–30 paid normal volunteers
Phase II	Determine the efficacy of the drug on the target disease under highly controlled conditions	Hundreds of patients with the target disease
Phase III	Determine the efficacy of the drug on the target disease under conditions of typical use	Hundreds to thousands of patients
Marketing for human use (requires approval of an NDA[2])		
Phase IV	Surveillance of toxicities reported during normal use	Patients

[1]IND: Investigational New Drug Exemption application requests permission to test the drug in human subjects.
[2]NDA: New Drug Application requests permission to market the drug.

3. Because they bind reversibly to the same receptors, partial agonists act like competitive pharmacologic antagonists when combined with full agonists.

IV. Drug Development and Regulation

A. In the United States, the **Food and Drug Administration (FDA)** is the government agency that mandates the conditions under which drugs intended for medical use are developed, tested, and marketed.

B. **Drug testing** follows a pattern of animal tests and human trials (Table 1–2).

C. In the United States, **prescription drugs** are drugs that are deemed to require complex directions regarding their use.
   1. They can be purchased only with a prescriber's direction (the prescription).
   2. Simpler and safer drugs may be marketed for sale without a prescription and are called **over-the-counter drugs.**

D. In the United States, **scheduled drugs** are drugs that are considered to have significant potential for illicit use (due to addiction liability and other reasons).
   1. Scheduled drugs are ranked according to their perceived social danger.
   2. Schedule I drugs are banned from prescription or anything other than research use.
   3. Schedule II drugs include strongly addicting drugs (eg, strong opioids and strong stimulants) that nevertheless have important medical uses.
   4. Schedule III, IV, and V drugs include drugs that are progressively less addicting.

CLINICAL PROBLEMS

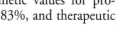

A 35-kg child with heart disease requires immediate treatment with the antiarrhythmic drug procainamide. The textbook lists the following pharmacokinetic values for procainamide in a 70-kg person: V_d 130 L, Cl 36 L/h, oral availability 83%, and therapeutic concentration 5 mg/L.

1. What intravenous loading dose should be administered?
   A. 180 mg
   B. 225 mg
   C. 270 mg
   D. 325 mg
   E. 783 mg

2. What constant intravenous infusion rate should be used to maintain the therapeutic concentration of 5 mg/L?
   A. 90 mg/h
   B. 108 mg/h
   C. 180 mg/h
   D. 217 mg/h
   E. 650 mg/h

3. What is the predicted half-life of procainamide in this child?

   A. 2.1 hours

   B. 2.5 hours

   C. 3.6 hours

   D. 5.0 hours

   E. 10 hours

A new drug has been developed by a drug company for outpatient use in hypertension. The animal tests of this drug resulted in the dose–response curves shown in Figure 1–8.

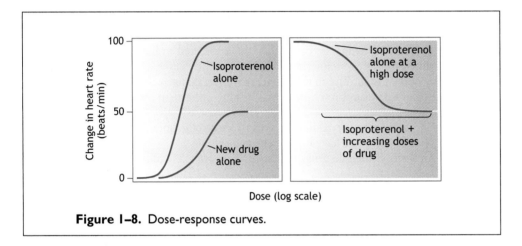

Figure 1–8. Dose-response curves.

4. Which of the following terms best describes the new drug?

   A. Full competitive pharmacologic antagonist

   B. Irreversible pharmacologic antagonist

   C. Partial competitive pharmacologic agonist

   D. Physiologic antagonist

   E. Chemical antagonist

5. Which of the following need **not** be accomplished before a drug can be tested in humans?

   A. Acute toxicity testing in animals

   B. Reproductive toxicity testing in animals

   C. Approval of an Investigational New Drug (IND) Exemption application

   D. Approval of a New Drug Application (NDA)

ANSWERS

1. The answer is D. This patient is half the weight of the average adult to whom the given pharmacokinetic values apply. Therefore the volume of distribution and clearance in this child will be approximately one-half of the given values. The drug will be given intravenously, so the oral bioavailability is irrelevant. The loading dose fills the volume of distribution so the dose required is

$$\text{Loading dose} = V_d \times C_p\,(\text{target}) = 130L/2 \times 5mg/L$$
$$= 325mg$$

2. The answer is A. To maintain a constant plasma concentration, the rate of administration must equal the rate of elimination:

$$\text{Rate of infusion} = \text{rate of elimination (at steady-state)}$$
$$= Cl \times C_P\,(\text{target})$$

In this 35 kg-child, Cl is 18 L/h, so

$$\text{Infusion rate} = 5\,mg/L \times 18\,L/h = 90\,mg/h$$

3. The answer is B. The half-life is determined by the ratio of V_d to Cl:

$$t_{1/2} = 0.693 \times V_d/Cl = 0.693 \times 130L/36L/h = 2.5\ \text{hours}$$

4. The answer is C. The dose–response curves show that the new drug has the same qualitative action as the full agonist isoproterenol on heart rate. The maximum effect of the new drug is less than that of isoproterenol, so the new drug is acting as a partial agonist at isoproterenol receptors (β adrenoceptors).

5. The answer is D. The NDA is the formal application for permission to market the drug for general medical use. It cannot precede the collection of the clinical data but is submitted after the clinical trials have been completed.

CHAPTER 2
AUTONOMIC NERVOUS SYSTEM PHARMACOLOGY

I. Autonomic Anatomy

A. The **autonomic nervous system (ANS)** controls involuntary body functions such as pupillary response to light, visual focus, blood pressure, digestion, and excretion.

1. The ANS contains both sensory (**afferent**) and motor (**efferent**) components.

2. The organs and tissues innervated include **smooth muscle, cardiac muscle, and glands** (Figure 2–1).

3. The ANS differs from the somatic (voluntary) motor system in having a **ganglionic synapse** in the efferent path.

B. The ANS is divided into the sympathetic and parasympathetic systems.

1. In the **sympathetic system,** the ganglia are located close to the spinal column, so that preganglionic neurons are short and postganglionic neurons are long.

2. In the **parasympathetic system,** the ganglia are located close to or in the innervated organs, so that preganglionic neurons are long and postganglionic neurons are short.

II. Transmitter Biochemistry

A. Parasympathetic Nervous System Neurotransmitters

1. **Acetylcholine** is the primary neurotransmitter in the motor limb of the parasympathetic system at both the ganglionic and postganglionic effector cell synapses.

2. Other substances found in transmitter vesicles [adenosine triphosphate (ATP) and peptides] function as **cotransmitters** when acetylcholine is released.

3. Acetylcholine is **synthesized** from **choline,** which is transported from the extracellular space into the neuron, and **acetyl-coenzyme A (AcCoA)**, which is synthesized in mitochondria in the nerve ending (Figure 2–2).

4. The acetylcholine is then **pumped into storage vesicles** by a carrier and remains in the vesicle until released by interaction of specific **vesicle-associated membrane proteins (VAMPs)** with cell membrane nerve ending proteins, known as **synaptosomal-associated proteins (SNAPs)**.

5. **Transmitter release** occurs when calcium enters the nerve ending and triggers an interaction between VAMPs and SNAPs, resulting in formation of a pore from the vesicle to the extracellular synaptic cleft. **Botulinum toxin** is an enzyme that cleaves certain VAMPs or SNAPs and thus prevents transmitter release from cholinergic nerve endings.

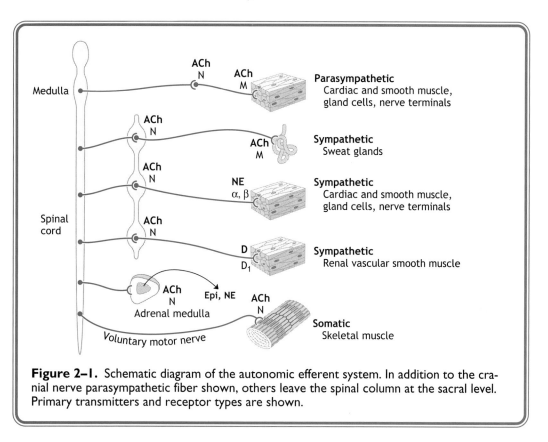

Figure 2–1. Schematic diagram of the autonomic efferent system. In addition to the cranial nerve parasympathetic fiber shown, others leave the spinal column at the sacral level. Primary transmitters and receptor types are shown.

6. **Termination of action** of acetylcholine occurs through hydrolysis of the transmitter by **acetylcholinesterase,** which is present in the synapse.

USE OF BOTULINUM TOXIN

Botulinum toxin is now available as a drug (**Botox**). It can be injected into localized areas to produce a controlled inhibition of acetylcholine release that is useful in alleviation of spastic conditions, reduction of facial wrinkles, and even control of excess sweating.

B. **Sympathetic Nervous System Neurotransmitters**
1. The transmitter at **sympathetic ganglia** is **acetylcholine,** but the transmitter at postganglionic effector cell synapses varies with the tissue being innervated.
2. For thermoregulatory sweat glands and some vasodilator fibers going to skeletal muscle blood vessels, **acetylcholine** is the transmitter released from the postganglionic fiber.
3. The processes of synthesis, storage, release, and termination of action for acetylcholine in sympathetic neurons are identical to those in parasympathetic fibers.
4. For most tissues, **norepinephrine (noradrenaline)** is the transmitter released from sympathetic postganglionic fibers.
5. **Synthesis of norepinephrine:** Tyrosine is pumped into the nerve ending cytoplasm by a carrier, hydroxylated to dopa (the rate-limiting step), and then converted to dopamine.

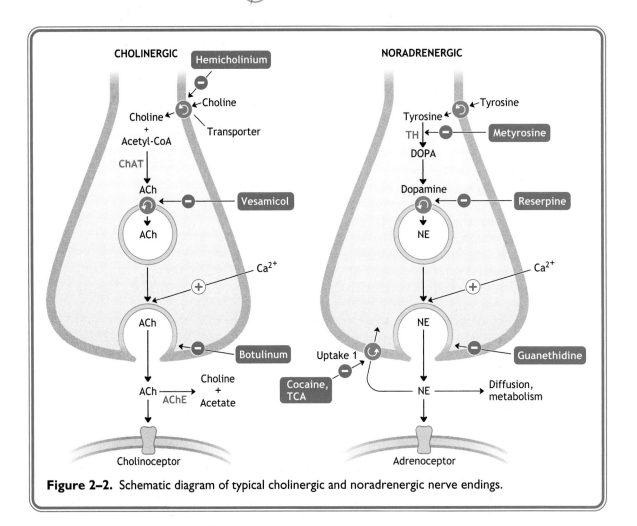

Figure 2–2. Schematic diagram of typical cholinergic and noradrenergic nerve endings.

    a. The **dopamine** is pumped into transmitter vesicles, where it is converted to norepinephrine (Figure 2–2).

    b. Hydroxylation of tyrosine can be inhibited by the drug **metyrosine.**

  6. Dopamine and recycled norepinephrine are **pumped into storage vesicles** where they are protected from the monoamine oxidase that is present on the mitochondria in the nerve ending.

  7. Norepinephrine is **released** from the nerve ending by an interaction of calcium with VAMPs and SNAPs, similar to that in cholinergic neurons.

  8. Norepinephrine is not metabolized in the synapse. Instead, its action is **terminated** by being taken back up into the nerve ending (**reuptake**) or **diffusing** out of the synapse.

NOREPINEPHRINE-SYNTHESIZING NEURONS AND BOTULINUM

Norepinephrine-synthesizing neurons *do not contain the endocytotic mechanism for taking up botulinum toxin. Therefore, unlike cholinergic neurons, they are not inhibited.*

III. Physiology of Autonomic Action

A. Receptor Types and Second Messengers

1. Transmitters released from autonomic nerves activate receptors on the postsynaptic cell membrane. The primary receptor types for acetylcholine and norepinephrine (and related agents) are listed in Table 2–1.
2. Muscarinic and norepinephrine receptors are coupled to effector enzymes and channels by **G proteins,** which translate the receptor activation into an enzyme effect appropriate for the particular cell type involved.
3. After activation of an effector enzyme by a G protein, **second messengers** [inositol 1,4,5-trisphosphate (IP_3), diacylglycerol (DAG), and cyclic AMP (cAMP)] are produced that bring about the further actions of the transmitter.
4. In addition to activating **postsynaptic** receptors, transmitters often activate **presynaptic** receptors (see Presynaptic Modulation, C.3, below).

B. Effects of ANS Activation

1. Activation of either division of the ANS usually results in multiple effects, sometimes involving the entire body (Table 2–2).
2. These effects provide important therapeutic targets for autonomic drugs. The usual mnemonics are:

Sympathetic effects: fight or flight
Parasympathetic effects: rest and digest

Table 2–1. Major receptor types for autonomic transmitters and related drugs.

Transmitter	Receptor Type	G Protein	Location	Effect and Second Messengers
Acetylcholine	Nicotinic	None	Ganglia	Opens Na^+, K^+ channel, depolarizes cell
	Muscarinic	G_q	Smooth muscle, some glands	Increases second messengers IP_3 and and DAG
		G_i	Cardiac muscle	Decreases cAMP, opens K^+ channels
Norepinephrine	α_1	G_q	Smooth muscle, some glands	Increases second messengers IP_3 and DAG
	α_2	G_i	Smooth muscle, preganglionic nerve endings, CNS	Decreases second messenger cAMP
	β_1, β_2, β_3	G_s	Smooth and cardiac muscle, juxtaglomerular apparatus, adipocytes	Increases second messenger cAMP

Table 2–2. Effects of autonomic nerve activity.

Organ or Tissue	Effect of Sympathetic Discharge (Receptor Type)	Effect of Parasympathetic Discharge (Receptor Type)
Eye	Dilates pupil (α)	Constricts pupil, focuses for near vision (M)
Airways	Dilates bronchioles (β_2)	Constricts bronchioles (M)
GI tract	Slows motility (α, β_2)	Increases motility, secretion (M)
GU tract	Contracts sphincters, mediates ejaculation (α)	Contracts walls of bladder (M), mediates erection
Vessels	Constricts arterioles in skin and splanchnic vessels (α), dilates in skeletal muscle vessels (β_2)	Little effect
Heart	Accelerates all pacemakers and AV conduction, increases force of contraction (β_1, β_2)	Slows sinus rate and AV conduction, increases AV refractory period (M)
Exocrine glands	Increases sweating (M), salivation (slight, α)	Increases salivation markedly, increases lacrimal, gastric, duodenal, and pancreatic secretion (M)
Metabolic effects	Increases glycogenolysis, free fatty acids in blood, renin release, and potassium release and uptake; potentiates thyroid effects (β)	Little effect
Skeletal muscle	Increases strength (α); causes tremor (β_2)	Little effect

   C. Integration of Autonomic Effects
   1. Integration of ANS action at one site with action at other sites is accomplished by several processes, the most important of which are organ-level compensation and local presynaptic modulation.
   2. **Organ-level compensatory processes** control the cardiovascular system, and to a lesser extent, the gastrointestinal (GI) tract and genitourinary (GU) tract.
      a. In the cardiovascular system, arterial blood pressure is precisely monitored by baroreceptor nerves. When changes occur (eg, due to a pressure-lowering drug) strong compensatory responses attempt to return the pressure to its previous level.
      b. These responses are mediated by the ANS and by the hormonal system diagrammed in Figure 2–3.
   3. **Presynaptic modulation** of transmitter release takes place through receptors on the membranes of nerve endings.

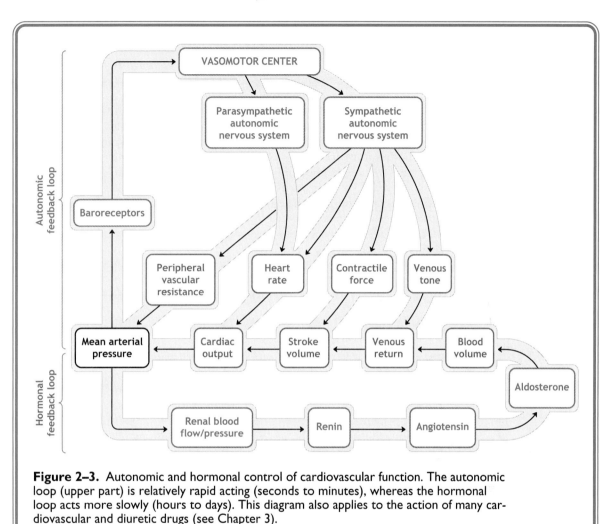

Figure 2–3. Autonomic and hormonal control of cardiovascular function. The autonomic loop (upper part) is relatively rapid acting (seconds to minutes), whereas the hormonal loop acts more slowly (hours to days). This diagram also applies to the action of many cardiovascular and diuretic drugs (see Chapter 3).

a. These receptors respond to the primary transmitter of the nerve and to many other substances. For example, nerve endings that release norepinephrine have been shown to contain α_2 adrenoceptors as well as muscarinic, histamine, serotonin, angiotensin, opioid, and other receptors.

b. These receptors may be positive or negative modulators, ie, they may increase or decrease norepinephrine release.

THE α_2 PRESYNAPTIC RECEPTOR

- *The α_2 **presynaptic receptor** has been studied in greatest detail because **clonidine**, an important antihypertensive drug, has its primary effect on it.*

- *Activation of this receptor **reduces** norepinephrine release.*

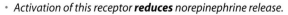

IV. Cholinomimetic Drugs

    A. **Mechanisms & Spectrum of Action**

        1. Drugs that mimic acetylcholine may act by two different mechanisms: by **directly activating cholinoceptors** or by **inhibiting acetylcholinesterase,** thus blocking the termination of action of endogenous acetylcholine.

            a. Like acetylcholine, **direct-acting cholinomimetics** may have affinity for both muscarinic and nicotinic receptors, or they may be more selective and activate only one of the two.

            b. **Indirect-acting cholinomimetics** (cholinesterase inhibitors) are **amplifiers,** which act only where acetylcholine is released from endogenous stores. As a result they have little or no effect at the uninnervated cholinoceptors that are present on the endothelium of blood vessels.

        2. Prototypes and related agents that are direct-acting and indirect-acting are listed in Table 2–3.

    B. **Actions of Muscarinic Cholinomimetics**

        1. **Eye:** The smooth muscle of the pupillary constrictor and the ciliary muscle is contracted. The pupil is miotic and the eye focuses for near vision.

        2. **Airways:** The smooth muscle in the airways is contracted. Wheezing may result.

        3. **GI and GU tracts:** The smooth muscle is contracted and motility is increased. Sphincters are usually relaxed.

        4. **Blood vessels:** The smooth muscle of most vessels has few cholinoceptors, but the endothelium lining the vessels carries many uninnervated muscarinic receptors.

            a. If these receptors are activated by a direct-acting cholinomimetic, the endothelial cells produce **nitric oxide,** a very potent vasodilator.

            b. The nitric oxide rapidly diffuses into the adjoining vascular smooth muscle and causes relaxation.

            c. **Blood pressure** may be significantly **reduced** and baroreceptor reflexes may be evoked (Figure 2–3).

        5. **Heart:** The heart is normally innervated by the vagus nerve, which causes **bradycardia** and slowed **atrioventricular (AV) conduction** when actively discharging.

Table 2–3. Cholinomimetic drugs.

Mechanism of Action	Receptor Affinity	Drugs
Direct	Both muscarinic and nicotinic	Acetylcholine, carbachol
	Muscarinic only	Muscarine, pilocarpine, bethanechol
	Nicotinic only	Nicotine, succinylcholine
Indirect	Little or none (binds to cholinesterase)	Edrophonium, neostigmine, physostigmine, parathion

      a. A similar effect results from indirect-acting cholinomimetics, which amplify these endogenous acetylcholine effects.

      b. In contrast, direct-acting cholinomimetics usually cause hypotension sufficient to evoke a strong compensatory **tachycardia.**

  6. **Exocrine glands:** Lacrimal, salivary, and thermoregulatory (eccrine) sweat glands are stimulated.

C. Actions of Nicotinic Cholinomimetics

  1. **Autonomic ganglia:** Both sympathetic and parasympathetic ganglia may be activated. Actions on dually innervated organs (eg, pupil and sinoatrial node of the heart) are unpredictable.

  2. **Skeletal muscle neuromuscular junctions:** Opening of the Na^+, K^+ channels on the end plate results in depolarization, and initially, contractions of muscle units. Maintained depolarization, which is caused by long-acting nicotinic agonists such as **succinylcholine,** results in block of impulse propagation from the end plate to the skeletal muscle membrane and leads to paralysis.

D. Clinical Uses

  1. The cholinomimetics have been used in the treatment of **glaucoma.**

      a. By constricting the pupil and contracting the ciliary muscle, they increase outflow of aqueous humor and thereby reduce intraocular pressure.

      b. **Pilocarpine** or **physostigmine** is applied topically to reduce systemic toxicity.

  2. Cholinomimetics are used in the treatment of **ileus,** a loss of peristaltic activity that may follow abdominal surgery or neurologic injury.

      a. The drugs cause a predictable increase in motility, but care must be taken to rule out obstruction before the drugs are given.

      b. **Bethanechol** or **neostigmine** is given orally or subcutaneously.

  3. **Urinary retention** is another complication of surgery or neurologic injury that may be treated with cholinomimetics. If obstruction is ruled out, bethanechol or neostigmine is satisfactory therapy.

  4. **Myasthenia gravis** is an autoimmune disease in which the nicotinic receptors of skeletal muscle are progressively destroyed, resulting in severe muscle weakness.

      a. Increasing the activity of endogenous acetylcholine combats the weakness.

      b. **Edrophonium,** the shortest acting of the cholinesterase inhibitors (15 minutes), is sometimes used to diagnose the condition because when given parenterally, it produces a prompt and highly diagnostic increase in voluntary muscle strength.

      c. Longer-acting cholinesterase inhibitors (**neostigmine,** about 4 hours, or **pyridostigmine,** about 8 hours) given orally are used for long-term therapy.

      d. The direct-acting cholinomimetics are of no value in treating myasthenia gravis.

TREATMENT OF MYASTHENIA GRAVIS AND GLAUCOMA

- *Myasthenia gravis, a rare disease, requires the use of indirect-acting cholinomimetics, which are life-saving. Immunosuppressant drugs are also important.*
- *Glaucoma is a common disease in the elderly that is usually treated with β blockers, prostaglandins, or nonpharmacologic therapies. Cholinomimetics can be used but are no longer first-line drugs for treating this condition.*

5. **Other uses:** Cholinesterase inhibitors, especially **organophosphate inhibitors** (eg, parathion), are widely used as insecticides in agriculture. Exposure of farm workers to these agents can cause serious toxicity.

E. **Toxicity**

1. The toxicities of direct-acting and indirect-acting cholinomimetics are similar, but because cholinesterase inhibitors amplify the nicotinic as well as the muscarinic actions of endogenous acetylcholine, more nicotinic manifestations may be observed. These toxicities are best remembered with the mnemonic **DUMBBELSS.**

   D **diarrhea, defecation** (a **muscarinic** effect)

   U **urination** (a **muscarinic** effect)

   M **miosis** (constriction of the pupils, a **muscarinic** effect)

   B **bronchospasm** (a **muscarinic** effect)

   B **bradycardia** (a **muscarinic** effect)

   E **excitation** [of the central nervous system (CNS) and skeletal muscle **nicotinic** receptors, followed by postexcitatory depression or block]

   L **lacrimation** (a **muscarinic** effect)

   S **salivation** (a **muscarinic** effect)

   S **sweating** (a **muscarinic** effect)

2. Exposure to powerful cholinesterase-inhibiting insecticides, such as **parathion,** may be rapidly fatal and prompt recognition and treatment are essential.

V. **Cholinolytic Drugs & Pralidoxime**

A. **Mechanisms & Spectrum of Action**

1. **Muscarinic receptor blockers** are competitive pharmacologic antagonists that shift the graded dose–response curve for agonists to the right. **Atropine** is the prototype drug (Table 2–4) and several other agents are in clinical use.

ANTIMUSCARINIC OVERDOSE

CLINICAL CORRELATION

*Overdose with **antimuscarinic drugs** such as atropine is usually treated symptomatically. If drug treatment is required, the **antidote** usually used is the cholinesterase inhibitor **physostigmine.***

2. **Nicotinic receptor blockers** include two separate groups of drugs that selectively block ganglia or the neuromuscular junction in skeletal muscle.

   a. Ganglion blockers are rarely used but neuromuscular blockers (Chapter 5) are very important in modern anesthesiology.

   b. Nicotinic blocking agents act as competitive pharmacologic antagonists.

B. **Actions & Toxicities of Muscarinic Blockers**

1. **CNS:** At **therapeutic doses,** muscarinic blockers cause sedation, some reduction of motion sickness, and reduction of parkinsonian tremor. At **toxic doses,** they may cause hallucinations or convulsions.

2. **Eye:** These drugs cause marked mydriasis and cycloplegia. Even at low doses, patients with glaucoma may experience a dangerous increase in intraocular pressure.

3. **Airways:** Muscarinic blocking agents have little effect on normal airways, but bronchospasm can be reduced in some patients with asthma.

4. **GI tract:** High therapeutic doses can reduce hypermotility and secretion of gastric acid, but other drugs are preferred. Salivation is markedly reduced by small doses.

Table 2–4. Some representative antimuscarinic drugs.

Drug	Properties	Uses
Atropine	Lipid soluble, enters CNS and eye readily, duration of action 4–8 hours except eye, > 72 hours	Reduces airway secretions and AV block; causes mydriasis and cycloplegia; an important antidote for cholinomimetic overdose
Scopolamine	Similar to atropine, strong anti–motion-sickness effect	Reduces motion sickness; causes mydriasis and cycloplegia
Benztropine	Enters CNS readily	Treat parkinsonism
Glycopyrrolate	Enters CNS poorly, good peripheral muscarinic blockade	Reduces parasympathetic effects on the GI and GU tracts
Ipratropium	Enters CNS poorly, short half-life in blood	Used by inhalation route for asthma
Oxybutynin	Enters CNS but strong peripheral muscarinic blockade	Reduces bladder urgency, spasm

    5. GU tract: Moderate doses reduce bladder tone and may precipitate urinary retention, especially in older men.

    6. Cardiovascular system: At therapeutic doses there is no effect on vessels, but heart rate and AV conduction velocity usually increase due to vagal blockade. At high doses flushing of the skin (by an unknown mechanism) may occur.

  C. Actions & Toxicities of Nicotinic Blockers (Table 2–5)

    1. Although **ganglion blockers** enter the CNS poorly and have little or no effect at the neuromuscular junction, they block both sympathetic and parasympathetic ganglia and therefore have widespread autonomic actions.

      a. Because they markedly reduce blood pressure, their primary use was in the treatment of hypertension.

      b. However, because of their very poorly tolerated autonomic toxicities (cycloplegia, orthostatic hypotension, constipation, urinary retention, and sexual dysfunction), they are rarely used.

    2. Neuromuscular blockers have two modes of action: competitive pharmacologic **antagonism** of acetylcholine or prolonged acetylcholinelike **agonist** action (see also Table 5–7).

      a. The antagonists, also known as **nondepolarizing blockers,** prevent normal depolarization of the end plate and can be surmounted by increasing acetylcholine concentration in the synapse (eg, with cholinesterase inhibitors).

        (1) These agents are widely used for surgical procedures of medium and long duration.

        (2) The toxicities of the nondepolarizing blockers consist of hypotension (from histamine release and ganglion blockade) and excessive neuromuscular block requiring prolonged respiratory support.

Table 2–5. Properties of some nicotinic-blocking drugs.

Drug	Properties	Uses
Hexamethonium	Prototype ganglion blocker, no CNS effects	None (obsolete antihypertensive)
Trimethaphan	Very short-acting ganglion blocker, parenteral only	Used in hypertensive emergencies
d-Tubocurarine	Long-acting (30–60 minutes) nondepolarizing neuromuscular blocker prototype, histamine releaser and weak ganglion blocker; requires good renal function for elimination	Produces neuromuscular paralysis for surgery; mechanical ventilation is usually required
Succinylcholine	An **agonist** that causes depolarizing neuromuscular blockade, very short (3–10 minutes) duration of action	Produces neuromuscular paralysis of very short duration

    b. Succinylcholine, a **depolarizing blocker,** is an agonist that causes **prolonged** depolarization of the neuromuscular end plate, blocking impulse conduction into the muscle membrane and resulting in paralysis.

        (1) The depolarizing phase (phase I) cannot be surmounted or reversed.

        (2) After a variable period, the paralysis produced by succinylcholine converts to a nondepolarizing type (phase II) and can be reversed with administration of cholinesterase inhibitors.

        (3) The major use of succinylcholine is to facilitate intubation and other procedures of very short duration.

        (4) The toxicity of succinylcholine consists of increased intra-abdominal pressure, arrhythmias, and postoperative muscle pain.

  D. Pralidoxime: A Cholinesterase Regenerator

    1. Pralidoxime is used as an antidote in severe **cholinesterase inhibitor poisoning** caused by organophosphate insecticides. (**Atropine** is also used in all cases of cholinesterase inhibitor poisoning.)

    2. Pralidoxime, a chemical antagonist, has a very high affinity for the phosphorus atom in insecticides. It combines with the phosphorus, breaking the bond between the insecticide and the cholinesterase enzyme and regenerating the free enzyme.

    3. Pralidoxime is used by intravenous infusion during the first 24–48 hours after insecticide exposure.

    4. Toxicities: Overdose can cause muscle weakness.

VI. Sympathomimetics

  A. Classification: Direct & Indirect Action

    1. Direct-acting sympathomimetic drugs combine with and activate adrenoceptors (adrenergic receptors). Examples include the catecholamines **epinephrine, norepinephrine, dopamine,** and **isoproterenol.**

2. **Indirect-acting** sympathomimetics cause an increase of norepinephrine (or, in the CNS, dopamine) in the synapse, which in turn activates the adrenoceptors. This occurs by two mechanisms.

    a. **Amphetamines** and **ephedrine** displace transmitter from its stores inside the nerve ending.

    b. **Cocaine** and **tricyclic antidepressants** inhibit the reuptake of transmitter into the nerve ending after its release.

B. **Classification: Receptor Selectivity**

  1. Each of the three major families of **adrenoceptors** comprises several different receptor types.

    a. α **Receptors** are divided into two major families, α_1 and α_2. Prototype agonists are listed in Table 2–6.

    b. β **Receptors** are divided into three families, β_1, β_2, and β_3 (Table 2–6).

    c. **Dopamine receptors** are divided into five families, D_1 through D_5. Only the D_1 and D_2 families have been associated with major functions in peripheral tissues, but all five may play roles in CNS function.

C. **Organ-Level Actions**

  1. **CNS:** Unlike catecholamines, most agents that act indirectly, such as amphetamines, cross the blood–brain barrier.

    a. Indirect-acting agents produce a dose-dependent sequence of stimulant effects, ranging from mildly alerting and reduction of fatigue to a definite elevation of mood and insomnia, and to marked anorexia and euphoria.

    b. Although not fully understood, these CNS actions are probably more closely related to dopamine release than to norepinephrine release.

  2. **Eye:** Activation of α_1 receptors in the pupillary dilator muscle results in mydriasis.

  3. **Airways:** Activation of β_2 receptors results in bronchodilation.

  4. **GI tract:** Both α and β receptors mediate reduced motility.

  5. **GU tract:** α_1 Receptors mediate increased sphincter tone in the bladder and prostate; β_2 receptors mediate uterine relaxation.

  6. **Blood vessels:** See Table 2–7 for these effects.

  7. **Heart:** β Receptors (both β_1 and β_2) mediate increased myocardial contractility and increased heart rate. The net heart rate effects of sympathomimetics depend on the reflexes evoked by blood pressure changes as indicated in Table 2–7.

  8. **Other effects:** β Receptors mediate increased glycogenolysis and hyperglycemia.

    a. Blood insulin levels and free fatty acids increase.

    b. Hyperkalemia, followed by hypokalemia, and leukocytosis may occur.

    c. In skeletal muscle β_2 agonists cause tremor at most doses and α agonists may increase strength at high doses.

USES OF SYMPATHOMIMETICS

- **CNS:** *Amphetamines are used to treat* **hyperkinetic attention deficit disorder** *and* **narcolepsy,** *and to* **decrease appetite.**
- **Pulmonary and cardiac:** *Epinephrine is the drug of choice for* **anaphylactic shock.** β_2 *Agonists (by inhalation) are the drugs of choice for* **acute asthmatic bronchospasm** *and* β *agonists are occasionally used to* **increase heart rate.**

Table 2–6. Adrenoceptor subtypes in autonomic tissues and their properties.

Receptor	Prototypes	G Protein	Second Messenger	Effects
α—all	Norepinephrine, epinephrine, phenylephrine	Depends on subfamily	Depends on subfamily	Depends on subfamily
α_1	Midodrine	G_q	↑ IP_3, DAG	Smooth muscle contraction
α_2	Clonidine	G_i	↓ cAMP	Inhibition of transmitter release, smooth muscle contraction
β—all	Isoproterenol, epinephrine	G_s	↑ cAMP	Depends on beta subfamily
β_1	Dobutamine	G_s	↑ cAMP	Cardiac stimulation, increased renin release
β_2	Albuterol	G_s	↑ cAMP	Cardiac stimulation, smooth muscle relaxation, glycogenolysis, tremor
β_3	—	G_s	↑ cAMP	Lipolysis
Dopamine—all	Dopamine	Depends on subfamily	Depends on subfamily	Depends on subfamily
D_1	Fenoldopam	G_s	↑ cAMP	Vasodilation
D_2	—	G_i	↓ cAMP	Inhibition of transmitter release

- **Vascular:** α Agonists are used to decrease blood flow (to **reduce bleeding** and **congestion** and to **prolong local anesthesia**). Dopamine is used to **maintain renal blood flow** in shock. Midodrine is used to treat **idiopathic orthostatic hypotension.**
- **GU:** α Agonists are sometimes used to **reduce urinary incontinence;** long-acting indirect oral agents such as ephedrine are suitable. β_2 Agonists such as ritodrine and terbutaline are sometimes used to **suppress preterm labor,** although their value is controversial.

Table 2–7. Effects of some sympathomimetics on blood vessels, blood pressure, and heart rate.

Drug	Receptors	Effect on Vascular Tone in			Effect on Blood Pressure	Effect on Heart Rate
		Skin, Viscera	Skeletal Muscle	Kidneys		
Norepine-phrine	$\alpha_1, \alpha_2, \beta_1$	↑↑	(↑)	(↑)	↑↑↑	↓↓ (Reflex)
Epinephrine	$\alpha_1, \alpha_2, \beta_1$ β_2	↑↑	↓↓	(↑)	↑↑	Variable
Isoproterenol	β_1, β_2	—	↓↓	—	↓↓	↑↑↑
Dopamine	D_2 (β, α at higher concen-tration)	—	—	↓↓	↑	Variable
Phenylephrine	α_1, α_2	↑	(↑)	↑	↑	↓↓ (Reflex)
Albuterol	β_2	—	↓↓	—	↓	↑

Parentheses around arrows indicates a small effect.

D. Toxicities
   1. **Amphetamines and cocaine** have a **high addiction potential** and are scheduled drugs unless mixed with other agents. They may also cause **seizures.**
   2. All sympathomimetics may cause **arrhythmias** and **myocardial infarction.**
   3. In high systemic concentrations, α agonists may cause hemorrhagic **stroke;** in high local concentrations they may cause local **tissue ischemia** and necrosis.

VII. Adrenoceptor Blockers
   A. Classification & Spectrum of Action
      1. Most adrenoceptor blockers are selective for α or β receptors.
      2. Two drugs with combined action are discussed with the β blockers.
   B. α Blockers
      1. The α_1-selective blockers (eg, **prazosin**), and the nonselective blocker **phentolamine** are competitive pharmacologic antagonists; their blockade can be overcome by high concentrations of α agonists, which may result from the discharge of catecholamines from pheochromocytomas.
      2. The nonselective blocker **phenoxybenzamine** is irreversible in its mode of action and is therefore preferred in management of pheochromocytoma.
      3. α Blockers prevent smooth muscle contraction normally produced by endogenous or exogenous α agonists.

a. The major cardiovascular effect of α blockers is **decreased peripheral resistance** and **blood pressure,** often accompanied by **reflex tachycardia.**

b. In the presence of high concentrations of epinephrine, α blockers cause an actual reversal of the blood pressure response to the agonist: the normal hypertensive response (mediated by α receptors) is converted to a hypotensive response (mediated by β_2 receptors). This unique phenomenon is called **epinephrine reversal.**

c. In the GU tract, α receptors mediate contraction of prostate smooth muscle; α blockers are able to **reduce urinary obstruction** in men with benign prostatic hyperplasia.

USES OF α BLOCKERS

- *The α_1-selective blockers are used orally in essential (primary) hypertension and in benign prostatic hyperplasia.*
- *Nonselective α blockers are used almost exclusively in pheochromocytoma.*

4. **Toxicities:** All α blockers may cause **tachycardia,** the reflex response to the lowering of blood pressure, although nonselective α blockers cause a much more marked tachycardia than do α_1-selective blockers. **Phenoxybenzamine** and **phentolamine** may cause GI upset, and α_1-selective agents sometimes cause an exaggerated postural hypotensive response after the first one or two doses.

C. **β Blockers**

1. β Blockers are used in a wide variety of conditions and have been produced with a corresponding variety of properties. All β blockers in clinical use are competitive pharmacologic antagonists.

2. **Propranolol** is the prototype full antagonist β blocker.

3. **Pindolol** is the prototype partial β agonist and is used exclusively as an antagonist. **Atenolol** is a prototype β_1-selective antagonist.

4. **Carvedilol** and **labetalol** have both α- and β-blocking actions.

5. All of these drugs are active orally and have intermediate durations of action. Some are also used topically in the eye.

6. **Esmolol** is a parenterally administered very short-acting β blocker.

7. β Blockers have important organ level effects.

a. **CNS:** β Blockers often cause sedation or lethargy and reduction of anxiety.

b. **Eye:** β Blockers reduce secretion of aqueous humor. There is no significant effect on the pupil or focus.

c. **Airways:** β Blockers cause marked bronchospasm in patients with airway disease, especially asthma.

d. **Cardiovascular system:** β Blockers slow the heart rate and AV conduction and reduce myocardial contractility. This results in a very useful reduction in blood pressure in hypertensive patients.

e. **GI and GU tracts:** β Blockers have little effect.

f. **Other:** β Blockers reduce skeletal muscle tremor, glucose release from the liver, renin release from the kidney, and thyroid hormone effects.

USES OF β BLOCKERS

- *β Blockers are widely used in the treatment of hypertension, angina, and arrhythmias.*
- *Long-term use has been shown to reduce mortality and morbidity in patients who have had a myocardial infarction and in those with heart failure.*

- *Oral β blockers reduce familial tremor and stage fright.*
- *Topical β blockers are frequently used for the treatment of glaucoma.*
- *Intravenous and oral β blockers are useful in the treatment of thyrotoxicosis.*

> **8. Toxicities:** β Blockers can cause symptomatic cardiac depression (bradycardia, AV blockade, and diminished cardiac output) and in patients with asthma, severe bronchospasm. Chronic therapy may result in moderately elevated blood glucose, lipid, and uric acid levels. Symptoms of hypoglycemia (eg, from insulin overdose) are masked.

CLINICAL PROBLEMS

A teenager presented at his local dentist for extraction of an impacted molar. He had never had a dental procedure and was so nervous that the dentist was unable to administer the local anesthetic. The dentist therefore administered a sedative drug intravenously, which had an immediate calming effect. He was then able to give the anesthetic and carry out the extraction. There were no complications and bleeding was minimal.

When the patient was asked to return to the waiting room, he fainted upon standing. He immediately regained consciousness, but had a marked tachycardia whenever he tried to stand. After 30 minutes of rest his orthostatic symptoms resolved and he was able to leave.

1. What mechanism caused this patient to faint?

2. What drug effect from the sedative might have caused the fainting?

3. Which of the following drugs would be most suitable for oral use in patients who faint frequently when standing up?
   A. Epinephrine
   B. Isoproterenol
   C. Atropine
   D. Ephedrine
   E. Prazosin

A farm worker is brought to the emergency department following exposure to an organophosphate insecticide in the fields. He is wheezing and shows signs of severe bronchospasm.

4. Which of the following would **not** be expected as a sign of cholinesterase inhibitor insecticide poisoning?
   A. Mydriasis
   B. Increased salivation
   C. Increased bowel sounds
   D. Urinary urgency
   E. Skeletal muscle spasms followed by paralysis

5. Which of the following combinations of drugs should be used in the treatment of this farm worker?

   A. Atropine and epinephrine

   B. Epinephrine and isoproterenol

   C. Norepinephrine and propranolol

   D. Atropine and pralidoxime

   E. Pralidoxime and propranolol

ANSWERS

1. Fainting was due to inadequate cardiac output and perfusion of the brain. Transient fainting of this sort is most commonly due to **venous pooling**—pooling of blood in the dependent parts of the body and reduced venous return to the heart—when the subject stands.

2. Constriction of the arterioles and veins of the legs is an important postural reflex that is driven by the sympathetic nervous system when baroreceptors signal a drop in blood pressure. Blockade of α receptors in the vessels would prevent this important compensatory response. Because the cardiac β receptors are still functional, marked tachycardia is noted. The sedative drug probably had a significant α-blocking action. An example of such a drug is promethazine.

3. The answer is D. Patients with chronic orthostatic hypotension may have hypovolemia, which can be treated by use of hormonal drugs that increase salt retention, such as fludrocortisone. Patients with normal blood volume may have autonomic dysfunction, which is best treated with long-acting orally active α agonist agents such as ephedrine.

4. The answer is A. Patients with cholinesterase inhibitor poisoning exhibit the DUMB-BELSS syndrome (see text). The effect in the eye is pupillary constriction (miosis) not dilation (mydriasis).

5. The answer is D. Patients with cholinesterase inhibitor insecticide poisoning should always receive atropine and should usually also receive pralidoxime.

CHAPTER 3
DRUG THERAPY FOR CARDIOVASCULAR DISEASES

I. Hypertension

A. Antihypertensive Drug Groups

1. **Hypertension** has severe, often fatal sequelae, including **stroke, myocardial infarction,** and **renal failure.**
2. It is treated with four major drug groups: **diuretics, sympathoplegics, vasodilators,** and **angiotensin antagonists** (Figure 3–1).
3. These drugs are quite effective in lowering blood pressure, preventing sequelae, and prolonging life.

B. Diuretics

1. **Diuretics lower blood pressure** by at least two mechanisms: **reduction of blood volume** and **alteration of vascular smooth muscle tone** (see section V, on diuretics).
2. **Thiazides** (eg, **hydrochlorothiazide**) are often adequate for mild and moderate hypertension, but **loop diuretics** (eg, **furosemide**) are usually required for severe hypertension.
3. Thiazides are used orally, whereas loop diuretics are used orally or parenterally, depending on the urgency of the situation. For example, in malignant hypertension (severe hypertension with rapidly progressing organ damage), furosemide is given intravenously.
4. **Toxicities:** Toxicities are given in section V, on diuretics.

C. Sympathoplegic Drugs

1. **Sympathoplegic drugs decrease sympathetic discharge or its effects on the cardiovascular system** (Figure 3–2).
2. **Centrally acting sympathoplegics are α_2-selective agonists.**
   a. **Clonidine** and **methyldopa** are useful in **mild to moderate hypertension.**
   b. Clonidine and methylnorepinephrine (the active metabolite of methyldopa) activate α_2 receptors in the brain stem and reduce sympathetic outflow, thereby reducing cardiac output, and to a lesser extent, peripheral resistance.
   c. Clonidine is active as given, whereas methyldopa is a prodrug that must be converted in the central nervous system (CNS) to methylnorepinephrine. Methylnorepinephrine is stored in vesicles in noradrenergic neurons and released slowly.
   d. The duration of action of oral clonidine is 8–12 hours and that of the transdermal preparation is about 7 days.
   e. The duration of action of oral methyldopa is 12–24 hours.

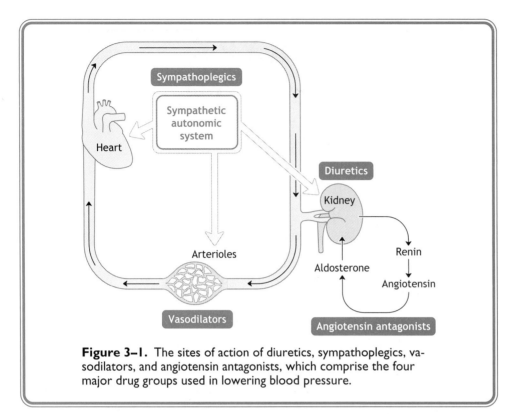

Figure 3–1. The sites of action of diuretics, sympathoplegics, vasodilators, and angiotensin antagonists, which comprise the four major drug groups used in lowering blood pressure.

  f. Toxicities: In ordinary antihypertensive doses, clonidine has minimal toxicity, but sudden cessation may cause severe rebound hypertension. The toxicity of methyldopa includes sedation, bradycardia, and rarely, hemolytic anemia.

 3. Ganglion blockers are **nicotinic cholinoceptor antagonists** (see Chapter 2).

  a. Trimethaphan is a rarely used parenteral agent for the **rapid reduction of severely elevated blood pressure** or for the induction of controlled hypotension (which is useful in some types of surgery).

  b. Trimethaphan blocks the nicotinic channel in autonomic ganglion cells and prevents synaptic transmission.

  c. The drug is given by constant intravenous infusion and the duration of action is 1–3 minutes.

  d. Toxicities: Trimethaphan may cause marked orthostatic hypotension, blurred vision, constipation, and urinary retention.

 4. Postganglionic sympathetic neuron blockers include **reserpine** and **guanethidine.**

  a. Reserpine and **guanethidine alter the storage and release of norepinephrine** and other amine neurotransmitters. They are rarely used.

  b. Reserpine blocks uptake of catecholamines and **5-hydroxytryptamine (5-HT)** into storage vesicles, thereby depleting transmitter stores in the nerve endings.

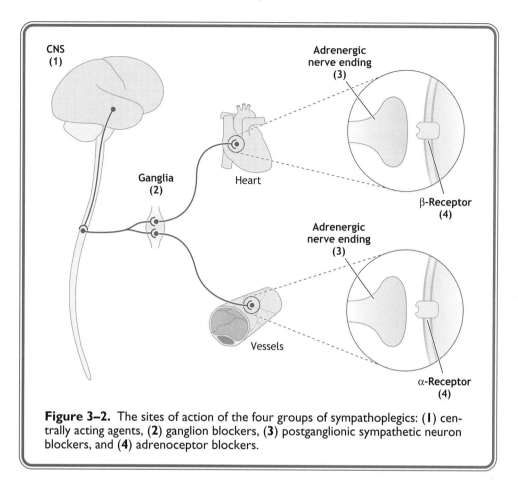

Figure 3–2. The sites of action of the four groups of sympathoplegics: (**1**) centrally acting agents, (**2**) ganglion blockers, (**3**) postganglionic sympathetic neuron blockers, and (**4**) adrenoceptor blockers.

    c. **Guanethidine prevents the release of transmitter vesicles** and secondarily also depletes norepinephrine stores.

    d. Reserpine is orally active, and has a duration of 12–48 hours.

    e. Guanethidine is also used orally, and has a duration of action of several days.

    f. **Toxicities: Reserpine may cause severe psychiatric depression,** so the dose must be limited; the drug should not be used in depressed patients. Reserpine may also cause diarrhea, nasal stuffiness, and sexual dysfunction. Guanethidine does not enter the CNS, but causes the same peripheral toxicities as reserpine, plus marked orthostatic hypotension and salt and water retention.

5. **α Adrenoceptor blockers** include **prazosin, doxazosin,** and **terazosin,** which are used for **mild to moderate hypertension.**

    a. These drugs selectively block α_1 **receptors,** causing a decrease in peripheral resistance.

    b. The selective α_1 blockers are orally active agents, with durations of action of 10–24 hours.

    c. **Toxicities:** Occasional marked first-dose hypotension, mild tachycardia, and salt and water retention may occur.

6. **β Adrenoceptor blockers** are extremely important as **monotherapy for mild hypertension** and as part of **polypharmacy for moderate and severe hypertension.**

   a. These drugs include multiple subgroups: **β_1-selective agents** (eg, **atenolol and metoprolol), drugs with reduced CNS effect (atenolol), partial agonist β blockers (pindolol), β blockers lacking in local anesthetic effects (timolol), drugs with some vasodilating action (carvedilol), and β blockers with a very short duration (esmolol).**

   b. Esmolol is used for hypertensive emergencies and acute arrhythmias.

   c. Except for esmolol (intravenous only), the β blockers are orally active; their duration of action varies from 6 to 24 hours (except for esmolol, which is active for 15 minutes).

   d. **Toxicities:** β Blockers may cause asthma, bradycardia, atrioventricular (AV) blockade, and heart failure. Less dangerous toxicities include mental lassitude, sleep disturbances, sexual dysfunction, and blunting of the response to hypoglycemia.

D. Vasodilators

   1. **Vasodilator** drugs are important as part of polypharmacy for **severe hypertension** (Table 3–1). The **calcium channel blocker subgroup** is also used in monotherapy for **mild to moderate hypertension.**

   2. **Hydralazine** is orally active and has a duration of action of 4–8 hours.

      a. **Toxicities:** Hydralazine causes moderate compensatory tachycardia (which must be prevented with reserpine or a β blocker) and salt and water retention (which must be prevented with a thiazide or loop diuretic).

      b. Hydralazine may also cause reversible systemic lupus erythematosus.

   3. **Minoxidil** is orally active and is converted to the active metabolite, minoxidil sulfate. Its duration of action is 4–5 hours.

      a. **Toxicities:** Minoxidil causes severe compensatory tachycardia (which must be prevented with a β blocker) and salt and water retention (which must be prevented with a loop diuretic).

      b. Minoxidil causes hirsutism and this has been exploited in a hair-restoring lotion preparation (Rogaine).

   4. **Balanced cardiac and vascular calcium channel blockers** include **verapamil** and **diltiazem,** L-type calcium channel blockers with similar efficacy in depressing cardiac and vascular smooth muscle.

Table 3–1. Mechanisms of vasodilator action.

Mechanism of Vasodilation	Drug Examples
Release of nitric oxide	Hydralazine, nitroprusside
Opening of potassium channels and hyperpolarization	Minoxidil sulfate, diazoxide
Block of L-type calcium channels	Calcium channel blockers (verapamil, diltiazem, nifedipine)

a. They are orally active, with half-lives of 6–7 hours.

    b. **Toxicities:** Both drugs may cause bradycardia, AV block, heart failure, constipation, and edema.

5. **Vasoselective calcium channel blockers** include the **dihydropyridines** (eg, **nifedipine**), which produce greater L-type calcium channel blockade in vessels than in heart.

    a. Dihydropyridines are orally active and have half-lives of 6–24 hours.

    b. **Toxicities:** Immediate-release nifedipine causes a sudden drop in blood pressure and compensatory sympathetic discharge. Dihydropyridines cause constipation and edema as well as (although rare) bradycardia, AV block, and heart failure.

6. **Parenteral drugs for hypertensive emergencies** include **nitroprusside** and **diazoxide,** which are used by intravenous administration.

    a. **Nitroprusside,** which spontaneously releases nitric oxide in the blood, is widely used in the United States, whereas **diazoxide,** a potassium channel opener, is used much less frequently.

    b. The duration of action of nitroprusside is a few seconds and a constant intravenous infusion is required. Diazoxide has a duration of action of several hours and can be given by intermittent injection.

    c. **Toxicities:** Nitroprusside may cause excessive hypotension and tachycardia; accumulation of metabolites cyanide and thiocyanate may occur. Diazoxide may cause tachycardia, salt and water retention, and hyperglycemia.

E. **Angiotensin Antagonists**

1. **Angiotensin-converting enzyme (ACE) inhibitors** (eg, **captopril and enalapril**) are useful as **monotherapy in mild and moderate hypertension** and are extremely beneficial in **heart failure** and in **diabetes.**

    a. These drugs **block angiotensin-converting enzyme,** thus reducing synthesis of angiotensin II from angiotensin I.

    b. They also **inhibit breakdown of bradykinin,** a vasodilator peptide.

    c. ACE inhibitors are orally active and **may be given once daily** even though their half-lives are much shorter (1–2 hours).

    d. **Toxicities:** ACE inhibitors cause cough, renal damage in nondiabetic renal vascular disease, and severe renal damage in the fetus (making them absolutely contraindicated in pregnancy).

2. **Angiotensin-receptor inhibitors** (eg, **losartan**) are used in patients who cannot tolerate ACE inhibitors.

    a. These drugs block angiotensin II AT_1-type receptors in the heart, blood vessels, adrenal cortex, and kidneys.

    b. Angiotensin-receptor blockers are orally active and have durations of action of 4–10 hours.

    c. **Toxicities:** The angiotensin-receptor blocking agents cause less cough than ACE inhibitors, but can lead to renal damage in the fetus; they are absolutely contraindicated in pregnancy.

PHARMACOLOGIC MANAGEMENT OF HYPERTENSION

• *Patients with **primary,** or **essential, hypertension** are initially given **monotherapy** (single-drug treatment), usually a **thiazide, β blocker, calcium channel blocker,** or **ACE inhibitor.***

• *Therapy is escalated to **polypharmacy** (multiple drugs) if monotherapy is unsuccessful.*

- *Drugs are chosen from different groups to maximize efficacy and minimize toxicity (eg, a diuretic plus a sympathoplegic plus a vasodilator).*
- ***Emergency,** or **malignant, hypertension** is associated with the risk of imminent myocardial infarction or stroke.*
  - *–Patients are **hospitalized** and treated with a **parenteral vasodilator, β blocker,** and **loop diuretic.***
  - *–Pressure is reduced gradually over a period of several hours, not suddenly, to prevent ischemic effects of reduced perfusion.*

II. Angina Pectoris

A. Types of Angina

1. **Angina** is a recurrent, severe, crushing pain in the chest, neck, or shoulder and arm that results from **myocardial ischemia** caused by **coronary blood flow that is inadequate for the needs of the heart** (Figure 3–3). Angina symptoms are often atypical in women.
2. It may occur when oxygen demand increases (**effort angina**) or when a coronary artery reversibly constricts (**variant angina**).
3. **Acute coronary syndrome** (**unstable angina**) signals an impending myocardial infarction and is treated as a medical emergency.

B. Nitrates

1. **Nitroglycerin, isosorbide dinitrate,** and other **organic nitrates** are useful in both effort angina and variant angina.
2. They are **venodilators that act through the release of nitric oxide** in smooth muscle of blood vessels.

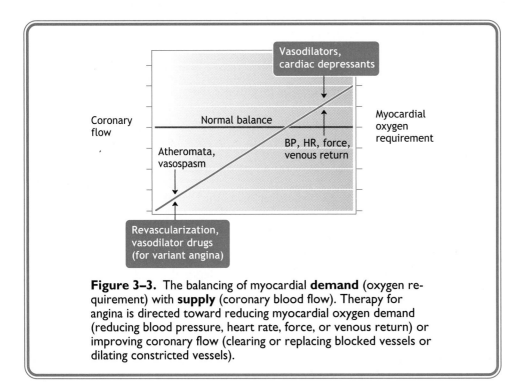

Figure 3–3. The balancing of myocardial **demand** (oxygen requirement) with **supply** (coronary blood flow). Therapy for angina is directed toward reducing myocardial oxygen demand (reducing blood pressure, heart rate, force, or venous return) or improving coronary flow (clearing or replacing blocked vessels or dilating constricted vessels).

Table 3–2. Effects of single drugs and combined drugs on variables that determine cardiac oxygen requirement.[1]

Variable	Nitrates Alone	β Blockers or Calcium Channel Blockers Alone	Combined Nitrate and β Blocker or Calcium Channel Blocker
Heart rate	*Reflex increase*	**Decrease**	**Decrease** or no effect
Arterial pressure	**Decrease**	**Decrease**	**Decrease**
End-diastolic pressure and fiber tension	**Decrease**	*Increase*	**Decrease**
Contractility	*Reflex increase*	**Decrease**	No effect or **decrease**
Ejection time	Reflex **decrease**	*Increase*	No effect

[1]Undesirable effects (effects that increase myocardial oxygen requirement) are shown in *italics;* beneficial effects are shown in **bold.**

3. Nitrates reduce venous return (**preload,** end-diastolic pressure), cardiac size, and diastolic myocardial oxygen consumption (Table 3–2).
4. They have lesser effects on peripheral vascular resistance and may reduce blood pressure (**afterload**).
5. Intravenous nitroglycerin is useful in acute coronary syndrome.
6. Nitrates are available in several formulations, including sublingual, oral, and transdermal patch.
7. Toxicities: Nitrates cause tachycardia, orthostatic hypotension, and headache. Transdermal nitroglycerin patch therapy is subject to development of marked tolerance if the patch is allowed to remain on the skin for more than 12 hours.

NITRITES

Nitrites *(note, not nitrates) are rarely used in angina but have found a medical application as antidotes for cyanide poisoning.*

C. Calcium Channel Blockers

1. Verapamil, diltiazem, and **nifedipine** and other **dihydropyridines** cause **smooth muscle relaxation** and **cardiac depression.**
2. They are used for prophylaxis of effort or variant angina, but have little or no benefit in acute coronary syndrome.
3. Calcium channel blockers act in effort angina by causing peripheral vasodilation (reduced afterload) and reduction of cardiac work.
4. In vasospastic angina they prevent coronary vasospasm.
5. Toxicities: Excessive cardiovascular effects (hypotension, AV blockade, and bradycardia), constipation, and edema may occur.

D. β Blockers

1. **β Adrenoceptor blockers,** such as **propranolol,** act to prevent angina by **reducing blood pressure** and **cardiac work.**
2. They are not effective in variant angina, but are very important in effort angina and acute coronary syndrome.

III. Heart Failure

A. Pathophysiology

1. **Heart failure (HF)** is a progressive and highly lethal disease that may follow uncontrolled hypertension, myocardial infarction, valve dysfunction, viral myocarditis, and other conditions.
2. The primary manifestations include **reduced cardiac output** and unfavorable compensatory responses such as **excessive sympathetic discharge** and **salt and water retention** (Figure 3–4).
3. Long-term changes include **remodeling, cardiac hypertrophy,** and cardiac cell **apoptosis.**
4. Periods of acute decompensation complicate longer periods of slow decline in cardiac function.

B. Diuretics

1. **Diuretics** are useful in almost all cases of HF (Table 3–3).
2. **Loop diuretics** (eg, furosemide) are particularly effective in acute pulmonary edema and in severe chronic HF.
3. **Thiazides** (eg, hydrochlorothiazide) may be adequate in mild chronic failure.
4. **Spironolactone** has been shown to reduce morbidity and mortality (see section V, on diuretics).

C. Angiotensin-Converting Enzyme Antagonists

1. **ACE inhibitors** (eg, **captopril**) reduce morbidity and mortality in patients with severe chronic failure.
2. They are first-line agents (along with diuretics) in HF and are used orally. Angiotensin II–receptor antagonists (eg, **losartan**) are used if ACE inhibitors are not tolerated.
3. These drugs reduce remodeling and sympathetic excess in chronic HF. They have little or no effect on cardiac contractility or the manifestations of acute decompensation.
4. **Toxicities:** ACE inhibitors cause cough and renal damage in the fetus, and thus are contraindicated in pregnancy (see section I, on hypertension).

D. β Adrenoceptor Blockers

1. Certain **β blockers** (eg, **carvedilol and metoprolol**) have been shown to prolong life in chronic HF. They are used orally.
2. The mechanism of action of β blockers in HF is unclear. It may involve reduced renin and angiotensin production and decreased apoptosis of cardiac cells.
3. **Toxicities:** β Blockers may cause worsening of HF, AV blockade, hypotension, and sedation.

E. β Adrenoceptor Agonist and Dopamine

1. **Dobutamine** is a **β_1-selective agonist** given parenterally for severe acute heart failure. Because the duration of action is short (minutes), dobutamine must be given by intravenous infusion. Although it is not β_1-selective, **dopamine** has similar benefits and toxicities in acute failure.

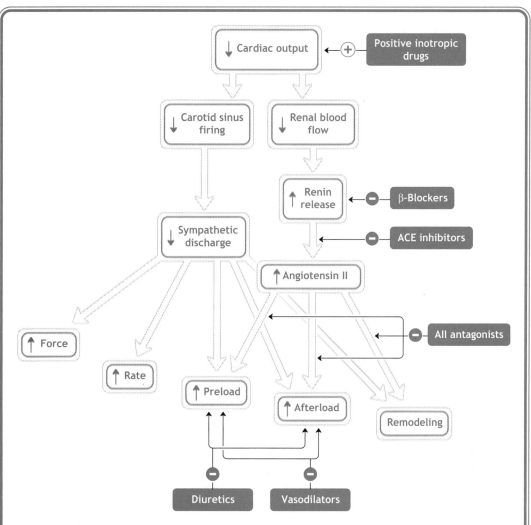

Figure 3–4. Pathophysiologic processes and drug targets in heart failure. Activation of the sympathetic nervous system and the renin–angiotensin–aldosterone system initially compensates for diminished cardiac performance, but thereafter accelerates the process of cardiac failure. Drugs that interfere with these compensatory responses are useful in therapy. β blockers probably have several additional sites of action.

   2. Dobutamine and dopamine increase cardiac force and reduce afterload, resulting in an increase in cardiac output.
   3. Toxicities: These drugs can cause tachycardia, arrhythmias, and angina.
F. **Cardiac Glycosides**
   1. Cardiac glycosides are steroidal molecules from *Digitalis* and other plants. **Digoxin** is the only important cardiac glycoside used in the United States.

Table 3–3. Treatment of heart failure.

Drug Group	Drugs	Beneficial Effects
Chronic failure	**(oral)**	
Diuretics	Thiazides, furosemide, spironolactone	Reduced preload, afterload; spironolactone, reduced aldosterone effects
Cardiac glycoside	Digoxin	Positive inotropic effect
Vasodilators	Hydralazine, isosorbide dinitrate	Reduced preload, afterload
Angiotensin antagonists	Captopril, losartan	Reduced remodeling, preload, afterload, apoptosis
β Blockers	Carvedilol, metoprolol	Reduced afterload, reduced remodeling, apoptosis
Acute failure	**(parenteral)**	
Diuretics	Furosemide	Reduced pulmonary vascular pressures, preload
β_1 Agonists	Dobutamine	Increased cardiac force, output
Vasodilators	Nitroprusside, nitroglycerin	Reduced preload, afterload

2. Digoxin, used primarily for HF, **blocks Na⁺,K⁺-ATPase** and increases intracellular sodium.
   a. The decreased outside/inside sodium gradient results in less expulsion of calcium from the cell and increased calcium stores in the sarcoplasmic reticulum.
   b. An increased release of calcium then occurs and causes increased contractility.
3. Digoxin also has a **cardiac parasympathomimetic effect** that reduces AV conduction. This action is useful in atrial fibrillation.
4. Digoxin is available in oral and intravenous preparations. Its half-life is 36 hours.
5. **Toxicities:** Cardiac glycosides are very toxic. They cause **cardiac arrhythmias, GI upset,** and rarely, neuroendocrine effects. Severe overdose causes cardiac arrest; this lethal poisoning must be treated with **digoxin antibodies** (Digibind).

G. **Phosphodiesterase Inhibitors**

1. **Amrinone, milrinone, aminophylline,** and **theophylline** are occasionally used parenterally for acute decompensation in HF. Their duration of action varies from 2 to 8 hours.

2. These drugs inhibit **phosphodiesterase** (**PDE**) and thereby increase the amount of cAMP in cardiac tissue and vessels.

3. **Toxicities:** The primary toxicity of PDE inhibitors is cardiac **arrhythmias.** Aminophylline and theophylline can also cause seizures. Because of these toxicities, PDE inhibitors are infrequently used in HF.

H. **Vasodilators**

1. **Nitroprusside** and **nitroglycerin** are administered intravenously for acute decompensation. **Nesiritide** is a newer vasodilator that also has diuretic properties. It is a peptide and is used intravenously in acute heart failure. **Isosorbide dinitrate** and **hydralazine** are occasionally used orally for chronic HF.

2. **Vasodilators** reduce afterload (increasing ejection fraction) and preload (reducing myocardial oxygen requirement) (see section I, on hypertension, and section II, on angina pectoris).

3. **Toxicities:** The nitrovasodilators cause orthostatic hypotension. All vasodilators can cause tachycardia. Nesiritide can cause renal damage.

HEART FAILURE

Heart failure is a common disease and has a high mortality rate. Therefore therapies that have been shown to reduce mortality (ACE inhibitors, some β blockers, and aldosterone-receptor blockers) are of major clinical importance.

IV. Cardiac Arrhythmias

A. Arrhythmias result from abnormalities of pacemaker activity or cardiac conduction.

B. Treatment includes electrical devices (pacemakers and defibrillators), electrical ablation of abnormal cardiac tissue, and drugs.

C. **Drugs for arrhythmias** (Table 3–4) are divided into five groups according to their actions.

1. **Group I drugs** act as **sodium channel blockers.**
2. **Group II drugs** act as **β adrenoceptor blockers.**
3. **Group III drugs** act as **potassium I_K channel blockers.**
4. **Group IV drugs** act as **L-type calcium channel blockers.**
5. **Miscellaneous drugs** include **adenosine, potassium ion,** and **magnesium ion.**

D. Three subgroups of sodium channel blockers are classified by their effects on **action potential (AP) duration** (Figure 3–5).

E. Electrocardiographic (ECG) effects reflect the actions of these drugs on action potential characteristics.

1. Group IA drugs slow intraventricular conduction (increased QRS duration) and increase duration of the ventricular action potential (increased QT interval).
2. Group IB drugs are highly selective for abnormal tissue and have little effect on normal sinus rhythm ECG.
3. Group IC drugs slow intraventricular conduction selectively (increased QRS duration).
4. Group II drugs slow AV conduction and therefore prolong the PR interval.

Table 3–4. Properties of the prototype antiarrhythmic drugs.

Drug	Group	Half-life	Route	PR Interval	QRS Duration	QT Interval	Toxicities
Adenosine	Misc	3 seconds	Intra-venous	↑↑↑	—	—	Flushing, hypotension, chest discomfort
Amiodarone	IA, III	1–10 weeks	Oral, intra-venous	↑	↑↑	↑↑↑↑	Corneal and skin deposits, thyroid dysfunction, pulmonary fibrosis
Disopyramide	IA	6–8 hours	Oral	↓ or ↑[1]	↑	↑↑	Antimuscarinic effects, heart failure, torsade[2] arrhythmia
Esmolol	II	10 minutes	Intra-venous	↑↑	—	—	Bradycardia, AV block
Flecainide	IC	20 hours	Oral	↑ Slight	↑↑	—	New arrhythmias
Ibutilide, dofetilide	III	6–7 hours	Oral	—	—	↑↑↑	Torsade arrhythmia
Lidocaine	IB	1–2 hours	Intra-venous	—	—[3]	—	Convulsions (rare)
Mexiletine, tocainide	IB	12 hours	Oral	—	—[3]	—	Convulsions (rare)
Procainamide	IA	2–4 hours	Oral, intra-venous	↓ or ↑[1]	↑	↑↑	Lupus (reversible), torsade arrhythmia
Propranolol	II	8 hours	Oral, intra-venous	↑↑	—	—	Bradycardia, AV block, heart failure
Quinidine	IA	6 hours	Oral, intra-venous	↓ or ↑[1]	↑	↑↑↑	Cinchonism, thrombocytopenia, torsade arrhythmia

(continued)

Table 3–4. Properties of the prototype antiarrhythmic drugs. *(Continued)*

Drug	Group	Half-life	Route	PR Interval	QRS Duration	QT Interval	Toxicities
Sotalol	III, II	7 hours	Oral	↑↑	—	↑↑↑	Torsade arrhythmia
Verapamil	IV	7 hours	Oral, intra-venous	↑↑	—	—	AV block, heart failure, constipation

[1]PR may decrease through antimuscarinic action or increase through channel blocking action.
[2]Torsade arrhythmia (torsade de pointes) is a very rapid polymorphic ventricular tachycardia.
[3]Lidocaine, mexiletine, and tocainide slow conduction velocity in ischemic, depolarized ventricular cells but not in normal tissue.

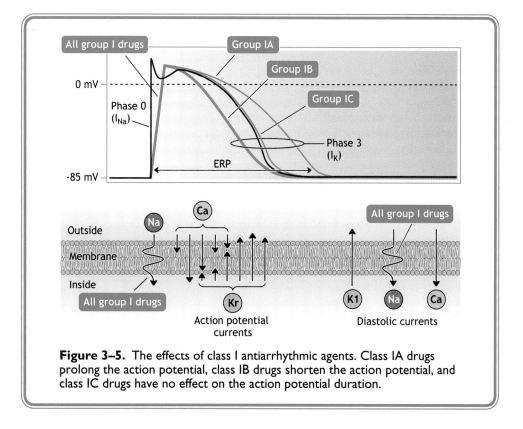

Figure 3–5. The effects of class I antiarrhythmic agents. Class IA drugs prolong the action potential, class IB drugs shorten the action potential, and class IC drugs have no effect on the action potential duration.

5. Group III drugs prolong the ventricular action potential and increase the QT interval.

6. Group IV drugs slow AV conduction and prolong the PR interval.

7. Adenosine markedly slows and blocks AV conduction and is used in AV nodal reentry arrhythmias. Potassium ion and magnesium ion are useful in arrhythmias caused by digoxin.

ANTIARRHYTHMIC DRUGS

*Antiarrhythmic drugs have a very low therapeutic index and can provoke new arrhythmias and heart failure. The Cardiac Arrhythmia Suppression Trial (CAST) showed that post–myocardial infarction patients treated prophylactically with group IC drugs had a 2.5-fold **increase** in mortality compared to patients who received placebo.*

V. Diuretics and Other Drugs Acting on the Kidney

A. Carbonic Anhydrase Inhibitors

1. **Carbonic anhydrase inhibitor diuretics** (eg, **acetazolamide**) are used as therapy for glaucoma and altitude sickness, and to reduce metabolic alkalosis.

2. These diuretics **block carbonic anhydrase** in the brush border and cytoplasm of proximal tubule cells (Figure 3–6) and in other tissues (eye and brain). Their effects on electrolytes are summarized in Table 3–5.

3. Acetazolamide is orally active. A few members of the group (such as **dorzolamide**) are available in topical form for glaucoma. These drugs have a duration of action of 8–12 hours.

4. **Toxicities:** Carbonic anhydrase inhibitors taken orally can cause gastrointestinal (GI) upset, paresthesias, and (in patients with severe hepatic impairment) hepatic encephalopathy. They are sulfonamides and are cross-allergenic with other sulfonamides.

B. Loop Diuretics

1. The loop diuretics (such as **furosemide** and **ethacrynic acid**) are used for conditions associated with moderate or severe hypertension or fluid retention (eg, HF, cirrhosis, and nephrotic syndrome). They are the most efficacious diuretics currently available.

2. These drugs **block an $Na^+/K^+/2Cl^-$ symporter** in the ascending limb of the loop of Henle. An indirect effect is to increase calcium and magnesium excretion in this segment of the nephron.

3. Loop diuretics are orally active but can also be used intravenously. Their duration of action is 2–4 hours.

4. **Toxicities:** Loop diuretics may cause hypokalemia, ototoxicity, and renal impairment. Their effects are diminished by nonsteroidal anti-inflammatory drugs. Except for ethacrynic acid, they are sulfonamides.

LOOP DIURETICS

Loop diuretics are very useful in the management of severe hypercalcemia. However, in this application an infusion of saline must accompany the diuretic drug to prevent hemoconcentration.

C. Thiazides

1. **Thiazides** (**hydrochlorothiazide** and others) are used to treat mild to moderate hypertension, mild heart failure, chronic calcium stone formation, and nephrogenic diabetes insipidus.

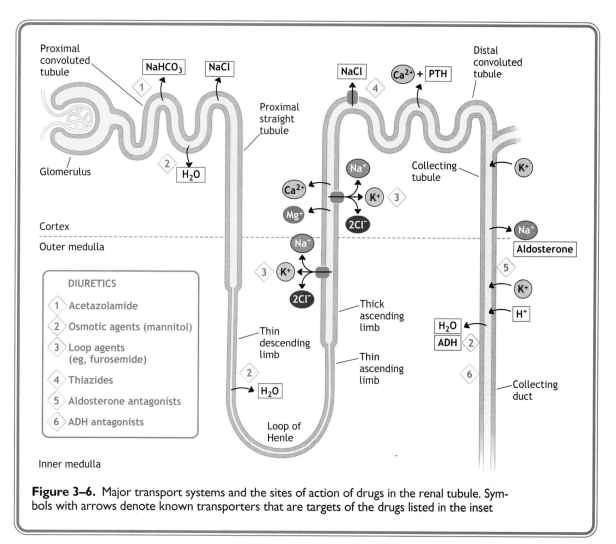

Figure 3–6. Major transport systems and the sites of action of drugs in the renal tubule. Symbols with arrows denote known transporters that are targets of the drugs listed in the inset

2. These diuretics **block an Na^+/Cl^- symporter** in the distal convoluted tubule. They increase calcium reabsorption and decrease its concentration in the urine.

3. Thiazides are orally active and are used almost exclusively by this route. Their duration of action is 8–12 hours.

4. **Toxicities:** The most important toxicity is potassium wasting. Thiazides may also raise blood glucose, lipids, and uric acid if used in high dosage. They sometimes cause significant hyponatremia. They are sulfonamides. Nonsteroidal anti-inflammatory drugs reduce thiazide efficacy.

D. Potassium-Sparing (Aldosterone Antagonist) Diuretics

1. **Potassium-sparing diuretics (spironolactone, eplerenone, amiloride,** and **triamterene)** are used for prevention of potassium wasting by other diuretics. Spironolactone and eplerenone are particularly effective in treating heart failure and other high-aldosterone conditions.

Table 3–5. Electrolyte changes produced by diuretic drugs.

Drug Group	Urine				Body pH
	NaCl	NaHCO$_3$	K$^+$	Ca^{2+}	
Carbonic anhydrase inhibitors	↑	↑↑↑	↑	—	Acidosis
Loop diuretics	↑↑↑↑	—	↑	↑↑	Alkalosis
Thiazides	↑↑	↑, —	↑	↓↓	Alkalosis
K$^+$-sparing diuretics	↑	—	↓	—	Acidosis

2. Spironolactone and eplerenone **block the cytoplasmic aldosterone receptor.** Amiloride and triamterene **block sodium channels** in the collecting tubule.
3. These drugs are orally active and have a duration of action of 12–72 hours.
4. **Toxicities:** The major toxicity is hyperkalemia. GI upset may also occur. Spironolactone has antiandrogen effects; eplerenone does not. These drugs are not sulfonamides.

E. **Osmotic Diuretics**
  1. **Mannitol,** the major **osmotic diuretic,** is used to treat acute glaucoma and to protect the kidney from solute overload caused by crush injury or chemotherapy.
  2. Because it is a small, nonresorbable molecule, mannitol osmotically inhibits the resorption of water in the water-permeable portions of the nephron.
  3. Mannitol is given intravenously and has a duration of action of 1–2 hours.
  4. **Toxicities:** Mannitol commonly causes headache, GI upset, hypotension, and mild hyponatremia followed by hypernatremia.

F. **Antidiuretic Hormone Agonists**
  1. In pituitary deficiency diabetes insipidus, **vasopressin,** or its analog **desmopressin,** is effective in restoring urine concentrating power to normal.
  2. In pituitary deficiency, the collecting ducts are responsive to vasopressin and insert additional water channels (aquaporins) into the luminal membrane to facilitate water resorption.
  3. In contrast, nephrogenic diabetes insipidus does not respond to pituitary peptides and must be treated indirectly with thiazides such as **hydrochlorothiazide.** Urine osmolality is increased but not to normal maximal levels.
  4. In nephrogenic diabetes insipidus, thiazides are given to decrease blood volume; this causes compensatory water reabsorption from the proximal tubule and reduces urine volume.
  5. The duration of action of vasopressin and desmopressin is 4–8 hours. Thiazides have an action lasting up to 12 hours.
  6. **Toxicities:** Vasopressin and desmopressin rarely cause vasoconstriction with hypertension or coronary spasm. The thiazides may cause hyponatremia, hyperlipidemia, and hyperuricemia.

G. **Antidiuretic Hormone Antagonists**

1. **Demeclocycline** is used to prevent dangerous hyponatremia in the **syndrome of inappropriate secretion of antidiuretic hormone** (**SIADH**).
2. Demeclocycline (like lithium ion) causes iatrogenic nephrogenic diabetes insipidus by blocking the action of antidiuretic hormone-like peptides.
3. Demeclocycline is used orally and has a duration of action of 10–16 hours.
4. **Toxicities:** Demeclocycline, like other tetracyclines, may cause disorders of developing bones and teeth in children. Rash, GI upset, and hepatic dysfunction are also reported.

CLINICAL PROBLEMS

A 55-year-old woman goes to a clinic because a health fair worker told her she had high blood pressure. She denies previous medical problems, but her parents died of cardiovascular disease (myocardial infarction and stroke) and one sibling is being treated for hypertension. Repeated measurements of blood pressure reveal an average of 160/105 mm Hg. Except for moderate obesity, the rest of the physical examination is negative. Routine laboratory tests indicate type 2 diabetes.

1. Which drug would be **least** appropriate for this patient?

   A. Captopril

   B. Diazoxide

   C. Diltiazem

   D. Hydrochlorothiazide

   E. Propranolol

2. Which drug would be **most** appropriate for this patient?

   A. Captopril

   B. Diazoxide

   C. Diltiazem

   D. Hydrochlorothiazide

   E. Propranolol

A 73-year-old man comes to his physician complaining of severe shortness of breath at night and swelling of the ankles. He has reduced his activity over the past year because of chest pain when he exerts himself. Physical examination reveals rales over both lungs, enlargement of the liver, and pitting edema of the ankles. Blood pressure is 140/90 mm Hg and heart rate is 95 beats per minute. His ECG is normal at rest. Cardiac enzymes and blood electrolytes are normal.

3. Immediate therapy should include which of the following?

   A. Atenolol and reserpine

   B. Furosemide and captopril

   C. Nitroglycerin sublingually and verapamil

D. Digoxin and diltiazem

   E. Dobutamine and hydrochlorothiazide

4. Which of the following drugs is most likely to prolong this patient's life?

   A. Captopril

   B. Digoxin

   C. Diltiazem

   D. Furosemide

   E. Nitroglycerin

5. Which of the following drugs is most likely to result in hypokalemia?

   A. Captopril

   B. Digoxin

   C. Diltiazem

   D. Furosemide

   E. Nitroglycerin

ANSWERS

1. The answer is B. Diazoxide, a parenteral drug, is inappropriate for this patient. It is not useful in outpatients with chronic hypertension and it is reserved for hospitalized patients with acute, severe hypertension. In addition, it often causes hyperglycemia, which would be very undesirable in a patient with diabetes.

2. The answer is A. An ACE inhibitor such as captopril is the antihypertensive drug of choice in a patient with hypertension and diabetes. These drugs are effective in many patients with hypertension and have been shown to prevent diabetic renal damage.

3. The answer is B. The major immediate problem is heart failure. Furosemide and captopril would be appropriate heart failure therapy. Atenolol or digoxin might be added later. The patient's secondary problem is angina of effort and it may be relieved by treating his heart failure. If control of heart failure does not eliminate his angina, then a β blocker or a long-acting nitrate such as transdermal nitroglycerin may be appropriate. Sublingual nitroglycerin may be appropriate for immediate control of angina attacks, but verapamil may exacerbate his heart failure.

4. The answer is A. Only three drug groups have been convincingly shown to prolong life in patients with heart failure. These are the ACE inhibitors, certain β blockers, and spironolactone. The drug of choice is captopril.

5. The answer is D. Diuretics that act in the proximal tubule, the ascending limb of the loop of Henle (furosemide), and the distal convoluted tubule may cause hypokalemia. Angiotensin antagonists (ACE inhibitors and angiotensin-receptor blockers) and aldosterone antagonists (spironolactone) cause hyperkalemia.

CHAPTER 4
DRUGS FOR ALLERGY, INFLAMMATION, AND BLOOD AND IMMUNE DISORDERS

I. Histamine and Antihistaminics

- **A. Histamine** is a **neurotransmitter** and **mediator of allergic responses.**
    1. It is synthesized from histidine (an amino acid) and stored in vesicles in mast cells, basophils, and some nerve endings.
    2. A metabolite of histamine, **imidazoleacetic acid (IAA)**, is increased in the urine of patients with **mastocytosis.**
- **B.** Histamine's effects are mediated by three **G-protein-coupled receptors** (Table 4–1).
- **C.** Histamine and other agonists at these receptors are of no clinical value but antihistamines are of great importance.
- **D. H_1-blocking drugs** (traditional antihistamines) fall into three groups (Table 4–2).
    1. The H_1 blockers are heavily used in the treatment of **hay fever** and **urticaria,** and a few other immunoglobulin E (IgE)–mediated allergic conditions.
    2. **Toxicities** reflect their autonomic nervous system (ANS) and central nervous system (CNS) effects (Table 4–2).
- **E. H_2-blocking** drugs such as **cimetidine, famotidine, nizatidine,** and **ranitidine** are very useful in the treatment of **acid-peptic disease,** especially **heartburn** and **peptic ulcer.**
    1. Because these agents are very safe, they are available over the counter.
    2. **Toxicities** (almost completely restricted to cimetidine) include inhibition of hepatic cytochrome P450 (CYP450) drug-metabolizing enzymes and an antiandrogenic action.
- **F.** No H_3-blocking drugs are available.

II. Serotonin and Related Drugs

- **A. Serotonin (5-hydroxytryptamine, 5-HT)** is synthesized from the amino acid tryptophan and stored in vesicles in **platelets, neurons,** and **enterochromaffin** cells in the **gut.**

Table 4–1. Histamine receptors and their functions.

Receptor	G Protein	Location	Function
H_1	G_q	Smooth muscle, gland cells, some nerve endings	Increased IP_3 and DAG[1], smooth muscle contraction (except vessels); increased secretion
H_2	G_s	Parietal cells (stomach), heart	Increased cAMP, increased acid secretion, cardiac stimulation
H_3	?	Nerve endings	Modulation of transmitter release

[1]IP_3, inositol 1,4,5-trisphosphate; DAG, diacylglycerol.

      1. An important metabolite, **hydroxyindoleacetic acid (HIAA)**, is increased in the urine of patients with **carcinoid tumor.**

      2. The effects of increased serotonin (and other substances) produced by carcinoid tumor include diarrhea, bronchospasm, variable changes in blood pressure, and flushing of the skin.

  B. Serotonin's effects are mediated by a large number of receptors, four of which are of clinical importance (Table 4–3).

  C. Serotonin is of no value as a drug, but two more selective agonist types are used.

      1. **5-HT$_{1D}$ agonists** (eg, **sumatriptan**) are useful in the treatment of **migraine** headache. **Toxicity** includes rare coronary vasospasm.

Table 4–2. Histamine H_1 antagonists.

Group	Examples	Uses	Toxicities
First generation, older	Diphenhydramine, dimenhydrinate	Allergy, sleep aid, motion sickness, nausea of chemotherapy	Strong α and muscarinic block; strongly sedative
First generation, newer	Chlorpheniramine, cyclizine	Allergy	Much reduced sedative and ANS effects
Second generation	Fexofenadine, loratadine, desloratadine, cetirizine	Allergy	Negligible CNS and ANS effects

Table 4–3. Clinically important serotonin receptors and their functions.

Receptor	Type	Location	Function
5-HT$_{1D}$	G-coupled	Neurons, other?	Mediates increased IP$_3$, DAG[1]
5-HT$_2$	G-coupled	Smooth muscle, other?	Mediates increased IP$_3$, DAG; smooth muscle contraction
5-HT$_3$	Ion channel	Chemoreceptors	Mediates nausea and vomiting
5-HT$_4$	G-coupled	Neurons in gut	Mediates increased gastrointestinal motility

[1]IP$_3$, inositol 1,4,5-trisphosphate; DAG, diacylglycerol.

TREATMENT OF MIGRAINE HEADACHE

CLINICAL CORRELATION

- *Acute migraine attacks are treated with simple analgesics, with sumatriptan or a similar "triptan" drug, or with ergotamine.*
- *Prophylaxis for severe recurrent migraine is partially successful using propranolol, amitriptyline, calcium channel blockers, and other drugs.*

   2. 5-HT$_4$ agonists (eg, **tegaserod** and **cisapride**) increase the release of acetylcholine in the gut and increase motility.
      a. This is valuable in conditions characterized by inadequate peristalsis.
      b. Toxicity of cisapride includes torsade de pointes arrhythmia, which has resulted in restrictions on the use of the drug. The major toxicity of tegaserod is diarrhea.

   D. 5-HT$_2$ antagonists (eg, **ketanserin**) have been developed for the treatment of patients with carcinoid tumor, but older drugs with overlapping effects (eg, **phenoxybenzamine,** a 5-HT and α blocker, or **cyproheptadine,** a 5-HT and H$_1$ blocker) appear to be just as useful. Ketanserin has been used to treat hypertension in Europe.

   E. 5-HT$_3$ antagonists (eg, **ondansetron**) are extremely useful antinauseant and antiemetic drugs for patients undergoing general anesthesia or chemotherapy.

   F. The **ergot alkaloids** are complex partial agonists at **5-HT, α adrenoceptors,** and **dopamine receptors.**
      1. Naturally occurring alkaloids include **ergotamine** and **ergonovine,** which are used to treat migraine headache and as an oxytocic, respectively.
      2. Semisynthetic ergots include **bromocriptine,** used in hyperprolactinemia and parkinsonism, and **pergolide,** used in parkinsonism.
      3. Lysergic acid diethylamide (LSD) is a semisynthetic ergot derivative with powerful hallucinogenic effects but no medical uses.

III. Eicosanoids

    A. **Eicosanoids** are products of a 20-carbon fatty acid, **arachidonic acid,** found in cell membranes. The two most important families of eicosanoids are the **prostaglandins** (**PGs**) and the **leukotrienes** (**LTs**).

    B. Prostaglandins are produced by the enzyme **cyclooxygenase,** which occurs as two isoforms, **COX-1** and **COX-2.**

        1. COX-1 is present in tissues in which prostaglandins are useful (eg, the stomach, where PGs protect the mucosa against acid).

        2. COX-2 appears to be more important in mediating pathophysiologic processes, especially joint inflammation.

        3. The nonsteroidal anti-inflammatory drugs (see section IV) are COX inhibitors.

    C. Leukotrienes are synthesized from arachidonic acid by the enzyme **lipoxygenase.**

Table 4–4. Actions of some eicosanoids.

Eicosanoid	Effects	Clinical Uses
Prostaglandins		
PGE_2 (endogenous)	Vasodilation, bronchodilation, oxytocic	Oxytocic (as dinoprostone)
PGE_1 analog misoprostol	Increased bicarbonate and mucus secretion in stomach	Prevention of NSAID-induced ulcers
PGE_1 analog alprostadil	Smooth muscle relaxation	Erectile dysfunction
$PGF_{2\alpha}$ (endogenous)	Vasoconstriction, bronchoconstriction, oxytocic	None
$PGF_{2\alpha}$ analog latanoprost	Increased aqueous humor drainage	Chronic glaucoma
Prostacyclin (PGI_2)	Prevents platelet aggregation, vasodilation	Severe pulmonary hypertension (as epoprostenol)
Thromboxane (TXA_2)	Facilitates platelet aggregation	None
Leukotrienes		
LTB_4	Leukocyte chemotaxis	None
LTC_4	Bronchoconstriction	None
LTD_4	Bronchoconstriction	None

1. The leukotrienes appear to be important in responses to immunologic challenge (eg, asthma and anaphylactic shock). Leukotriene inhibitors are used in asthma (see section IX).
2. The actions of some eicosanoids are summarized in Table 4–4.

IV. Nonsteroidal Anti-inflammatory Drugs and Drugs Used in Fever and Minor Pain and Headache

A. The **nonsteroidal anti-inflammatory drugs** (**NSAIDs**) are so-called to distinguish them from steroids (eg, prednisone; see Chapter 6): steroids have powerful anti-inflammatory actions, whereas the NSAIDs have weaker anti-inflammatory actions, but are more suitable for long-term therapy because they are less toxic.
   1. The older NSAIDs include **aspirin** and **salicylate.**
   2. Newer non–COX-selective NSAIDs include **indomethacin, ibuprofen,** and many others (Table 4–5).
   3. The selective COX-2 inhibitors are newer still and include **celecoxib** and **valdecoxib.**

Table 4–5. Properties of NSAIDs.

Drug	Half-life	Comments
Aspirin	15 minutes (but active metabolite has long half-life, see salicylic acid)	Converted to salicylic acid; wide use for pain, fever, inflammation, and antiplatelet action
Celecoxib	11 hours	Selective COX-2 inhibitor; a sulfonamide
Diclofenac	1.1 hours	General use in inflammation, pain
Ibuprofen	2 hours	General use in inflammation, pain
Indomethacin	4–5 hours	General use in inflammation, pain
Ketorolac	4–10 hours	Parenteral use in pain; an opioid substitute
Naproxen	12 hours	Longer action
Piroxicam	20 hours	Longest action
Salicylic acid	3–15 hours	Active metabolite of aspirin, zero order elimination at high concentrations

4. Aspirin is distinct from all other NSAIDs because it irreversibly blocks cyclooxygenase, especially in platelets. Its antiplatelet effect, therefore, is longer in duration (24–48 hours) than its anti-inflammatory and analgesic action (4–6 hours).

B. The NSAIDs are well absorbed after oral administration. Most are excreted via the kidney.

C. **Toxicities** of NSAIDs include gastrointestinal (GI) upset, peptic ulcers with or without bleeding, renal damage, and diversion of arachidonic acid metabolism to the leukotriene pathway. The latter effect may rarely present with the clinical picture of an allergic response to aspirin, including anaphylaxis.

    1. The COX-2–selective inhibitors have a lower risk of GI bleeding but are associated with an increased risk of cardiovascular events (myocardial infarction and stroke).

    2. Use of aspirin in children with viral infections has been associated with an increased risk of Reye's syndrome.

D. **Acetaminophen** has analgesic and antipyretic efficacy similar to aspirin, but is a very weak COX inhibitor and has little or no anti-inflammatory action. In overdosage, metabolites of acetaminophen can cause hepatic necrosis.

CLINICAL APPLICATIONS OF NSAIDS

CLINICAL CORRELATION

- *At low doses, **aspirin** is a very effective **antiplatelet agent** and is widely used to reduce the risk of myocardial infarction and stroke.*
- *At moderate doses, **acetaminophen** and all of the NSAIDs are effective **mild analgesics** for conditions such as **headache** and **muscle and joint aches** and also reduce fever. Most of these agents are also effective against **dysmenorrhea,** in which prostaglandins released from the endometrium play a major role.*
- *At higher doses, the NSAIDs (but not acetaminophen) are effective anti-inflammatory drugs and are heavily used for **arthritis.** Unfortunately, they do not slow progression of joint damage.*

V. Drugs Used in Gout

A. Gout is a chronic metabolic disease characterized by an elevated body load of uric acid and manifested by deposits of urate crystals in soft tissues and joints.

B. In the joints, these crystals trigger episodes of acute painful arthritis.

C. Three classes of drugs are used in the treatment of gout.

    1. Anti-inflammatory agents are the mainstay of therapy for acute joint pain.
      a. Ibuprofen and **indomethacin** are often used.
      b. Colchicine, a drug that inhibits motility of inflammatory cells in the joints by interfering with microtubule assembly, is highly selective for gouty arthritis.
      c. Colchicine is usually restricted to low-dose prophylactic therapy because of GI and hepatic toxicity.

    2. Uricosuric agents are effective in increasing the excretion of uric acid in the urine. **Probenecid** and **sulfinpyrazone** are used to inhibit the uric acid reabsorption transporter in the straight segment of the proximal tubule of the nephron.

    3. An **inhibitor of uric acid synthesis (allopurinol)** inhibits the enzyme xanthine oxidase and reduces the concentration of the very insoluble uric acid while increasing the concentration of the more soluble uric acid precursors, xanthine and hypoxanthine.

CLINICAL CORRELATION

TREATMENT OF GOUT

- *Acute attacks of gout require strong anti-inflammatory drugs, strong analgesics, or both.*
- ***Indomethacin*** *and* ***ketorolac*** *are NSAIDs with both properties that are often used for this purpose. Ketorolac may be used parenterally.*
- *Prophylaxis of gout may be carried out with uricosurics or allopurinol.*
- ***Uricosurics*** *may precipitate an immediate attack and should always be used in conjunction with* ***colchicine*** *or other agents initially.*
- ***Allopurinol's*** *benefits are relatively slow in onset and are suitable only for long-term therapy.*

VI. Antilipid Drugs

A. Hyperlipidemia is a cause of **atherosclerosis** and a major contributor to cardiovascular disease (**angina, heart failure, myocardial infarction,** and **stroke**).

1. The major lipids found in the blood consist of **lipoproteins** (macromolecular complexes of cholesterol, other lipids, and proteins) and **triglycerides** (fatty acid-glycerol esters).
2. In addition to cardiovascular disease, **hypertriglyceridemia** contributes to increased risk of **acute pancreatitis.**

B. Drugs used in hypercholesterolemia include **statins, resins, ezetimibe, niacin,** and **fibrates.**

1. The **statins** (eg, **lovastatin** and **atorvastatin**) are inhibitors of cholesterol synthesis, and the reduced intracellular cholesterol concentration results in increased production of low-density lipoprotein (LDL)–binding receptors on liver cells, which increases clearance of LDL particles from the bloodstream (Figure 4–1). Most statins reduce LDL cholesterol and have little effect on triglycerides, but atorvastatin reduces both.
2. The **resins** (eg, **cholestyramine** and **colestipol**) are nonabsorbable macromolecules that bind to and prevent reabsorption of cholesterol and bile acids from the gut (Figure 4–1). Reduced cholesterol returning to the liver stimulates the production of more LDL receptors and increased clearance of LDL particles. Resins tend to increase triglycerides.
3. **Ezetimibe** is a new drug that reduces intestinal absorbtion of cholesterol. Its mechanism of action is unknown.
4. The action of **niacin** (**nicotinic acid** and **vitamin B$_3$**) is not fully understood, but high doses cause a decrease in the secretion of very-low-density lipoprotein (VLDL) particles from the liver into the blood and decreased LDL formation (Figure 4–1). Niacin is also effective in **hypertriglyceridemia** and may increase high-density lipoproteins (HDL).
5. The fibrates (eg, **gemfibrozil** and **fenofibrate**) activate peroxisome proliferator-activated receptor-α (PPAR-α), which increases synthesis of lipoprotein lipase and other enzymes involved in lipid metabolism (Figure 4–1). **Serum triglyceride concentrations are reduced** and there may also be some reduction in LDL.

C. Toxicities of the antilipid drugs are varied.

1. Statins may cause serious skeletal muscle or liver damage and interfere with myelination in growing infants. These drugs are contraindicated in pregnancy.
2. **Niacin** in the high doses used for hyperlipidemia causes a transient uncomfortable flush with itching. Intensity of this reaction can be reduced with

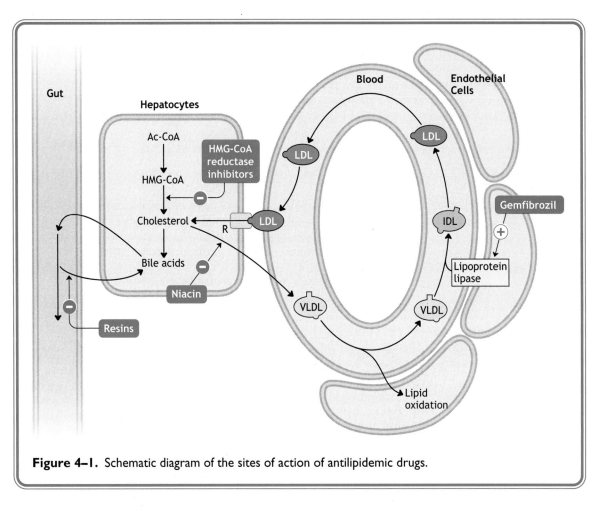

Figure 4–1. Schematic diagram of the sites of action of antilipidemic drugs.

aspirin. **Niacin** may also rarely cause elevation of liver enzymes, hyper-uricemia, and glucose intolerance.

3. **Resins** have an unpleasant gritty taste and cause GI discomfort, including bloating and constipation. Absorption of fat-soluble vitamins and drugs may be impaired. Resins should be avoided in hypertriglyceridemia.

4. **Fibrates** cause nausea, skin rash, and possible increased effect of antiplatelet drugs. The fibrates sometimes cause increased risk of gallstones.

VII. Anticoagulants, Antiplatelet Drugs, and Fibrinolytics

A. Anticoagulants include **warfarin,** an oral agent, and **heparin,** which must be given parenterally. Heparin is available in both high-molecular-weight (HMW) and low-molecular-weight (LMW) forms.

1. **Warfarin** acts by blocking the reactivation of vitamin K epoxide; it is a **competitive vitamin K antagonist.**

   a. Because vitamin K is essential for the hepatic synthesis of coagulation factors II, VII, IX, and X, warfarin causes a gradual depletion of active factors and inhibition of thrombin formation during the clotting process.

b. Warfarin's effects vary significantly among patients and must be monitored with the prothrombin time (PT) test.

  2. Heparin in its HMW form binds coagulation factor **Xa** and **antithrombin III.**

    a. Antithrombin III in this bound form is activated 1000-fold, so clotting is inhibited immediately on exposure to the drug.

      (1) Heparin is a large polymeric molecule of 12,000–30,000 MW that must be administered intravenously or subcutaneously.

      (2) Because of variable response, clotting must be monitored with the activated partial thromboplastin time test (aPTT).

    b. LMW heparins (eg, **enoxaparin** and **dalteparin**) consist of smaller-molecular-weight fragments (6000–15,000 MW).

      (1) These drugs inhibit factor Xa, but have less effect on antithrombin III than does HMW heparin.

      (2) They have a more predictable patient response and do not require regular monitoring of coagulation.

  3. The major **clinical applications** of heparins and warfarin are in the prevention and treatment of venous clotting, especially **deep vein thrombosis.**

  4. Toxicities: The major toxicity of anticoagulants is **bleeding. Warfarin is teratogenic** and cannot be used by pregnant women. **Heparin** causes a mild dose-dependent **thrombocytopenia** regularly, but occasionally causes a much more severe loss of platelets.

B. Antiplatelet drugs, which interfere with platelet aggregation, are particularly important in the prevention of arterial clotting as in **acute coronary syndrome** and **myocardial infarction.** The most important **toxicity is bleeding.**

  1. Aspirin irreversibly blocks the synthesis of **thromboxane** in platelets and provides a 24- to 48-hour effect at very low doses (<300 mg/d). Other NSAIDs have a similar but shorter and reversible effect.

  2. Clopidogrel and **ticlopidine** are oral drugs that irreversibly block the **adenosine diphosphate (ADP) receptor** on platelets.

  3. The **fiban** drugs (**eptifibatide** and **tirofiban**) and **abciximab,** a monoclonal antibody, competitively inhibit the binding of fibrinogen to the platelet IIb/IIIa receptor. The IIb/IIIa blockers are given parenterally.

C. Fibrinolytic drugs (Table 4–6) activate endogenous plasminogen to plasmin, an enzyme that breaks down fibrin and thus dissolves preformed clots.

  1. Unfortunately, plasmin may also degrade fibrin and fibrinogen in protective clots; therefore, the major toxicity of all the fibrinolytic drugs is bleeding.

  2. The most important clinical use is intravenous administration for **pulmonary embolism** and myocardial infarction.

VIII. Drugs Used in Anemias and Other Disorders of Blood Formation

  A. Anemia, a deficiency of red blood cell (RBC) mass or function, results from inadequate dietary iron, inadequate vitamin intake, inadequate RBC production, or accelerated RBC breakdown (hemolytic anemia).

  B. Iron deficiency anemia, the most common form, is effectively treated by supplemental dietary iron. Iron is irritating to the GI tract and in children can cause fatal poisoning.

  C. Megaloblastic anemia is caused by inadequate **folic acid** or **vitamin B$_{12}$** absorption.

Table 4–6. Fibrinolytic drugs.

Drug	Source	Cost	Toxicity
Streptokinase	Bacterial culture	Low	Allergic response; bleeding
Alteplase (tPA), reteplase	Recombinant DNA technology	Very high	Bleeding
Urokinase	Human cell culture	Very high	Bleeding

1. Folic acid can be readily absorbed from the gut, so simple supplementation of the diet is adequate therapy.
2. Vitamin B_{12} requires the presence of intrinsic factor for absorption.
3. In pernicious anemia and gastric carcinoma, synthesis of intrinsic factor is inadequate, so dietary supplementation of the vitamin is not very effective. In this situation, parenteral vitamin B_{12} must be administered, usually monthly.

USE AND TOXICITY OF IRON AND VITAMINS FOR ANEMIA

CLINICAL CORRELATION

- For simple iron deficiency anemia, oral supplementation in the form of **ferrous sulfate** or **ferrous gluconate** is effective. The ferric iron salts are poorly absorbed.
- Iron is irritating to the stomach and some patients cannot tolerate the doses required for rapid correction of severe deficiency. Parenteral iron (**iron dextran, iron sucrose complex,** and **iron gluconate complex**) is available for such patients.
- Because oral iron formulations are often used by women with young children, pediatric iron poisoning is an important problem. Manifestations include vomiting, abdominal pain, diarrhea, and necrotizing enteritis, followed by shock, lethargy, metabolic acidosis, and death. Prompt diagnosis and treatment with an iron chelator, **deferoxamine,** are essential.
- Folic acid and vitamin B_{12} are nontoxic. Folic acid is included in many "enriched" foods.

D. **Depressed blood cell production** can be treated with four different growth factors.
1. **Inadequate RBC production** is common in patients with chronic renal failure because the amount of the naturally occurring growth factor **erythropoietin** (which is secreted by the kidney) falls to an inadequate level. **Epoetin** is given in renal failure and in AIDS (Table 4–7). Inadequate production of RBCs, leukocytes, and platelets often occurs in patients given large doses of cancer chemotherapeutic drugs.
2. **Sargramostim (granulocyte-macrophage colony-stimulating factor, GM-CSF)** is a general growth factor for blood cell precursors.
3. **Filgrastim (granulocyte colony-stimulating factor, G-CSF)** is a more selective neutrophil growth factor.
4. **Interleukin 11 (IL-11)** is used to stimulate platelet production (Table 4–7).

Table 4–7. Growth factors used for anemia, leukopenia, and thrombocytopenia.

Condition	Drug	Effects	Toxicity
Anemia	Epoetin (human recombinant erythropoietin)	Increases red blood cell production	Hypertension, thrombotic events
Granulocytopenia	Filgrastim (human recombinant granulocyte colony-stimulating factor, G-CSF)	Increases neutrophil production	Bone pain
	Sargramostim (human recombinant granulocyte-macrophage colony-stimulating factor, GM-CSF)	Stimulates most marrow precursors but increases neutrophil production most	Fever, myalgia, peripheral and pulmonary edema
Thrombocytopenia	Oprelvekin (human recombinant inter-leukin-11)	Stimulates platelet production	Fatigue, headache, dizziness

IX. Drugs Used in Asthma

A. **Asthma** is characterized by transient episodes of **bronchoconstriction** superimposed on **chronic airway inflammation.**

1. Therapy therefore consists of **bronchodilators** for control of symptoms and **anti-inflammatory drugs** for prophylaxis (Figure 4–2).

2. Symptomatic bronchoconstriction in asthma appears to be mediated largely by the release of leukotrienes and other smooth muscle activators from mast cells and eosinophils in the airways.

B. **Bronchodilators** consist of β_2-**selective agonists, muscarinic blockers,** and **theophylline.**

1. β_2-**Selective agonists** (see Chapter 2) are the drugs of choice in acute episodes of asthmatic bronchoconstriction.

a. They act as physiologic antagonists against leukotrienes and other bronchoconstrictors by increasing cAMP in smooth muscle.

b. Agents such as **albuterol, metaproterenol,** and others are given by metered-dose inhaler as often as required to control symptoms.

c. Toxicities include tremor and tachycardia, but it is important **not** to limit the amount of the drug during an acute attack because uncontrolled bronchoconstriction can be fatal.

2. **Ipratropium** and tiotropium are atropinelike muscarinic antagonists.

a. They are available in metered-dose inhaler form, but are not as generally effective as the β_2-selective agonists.

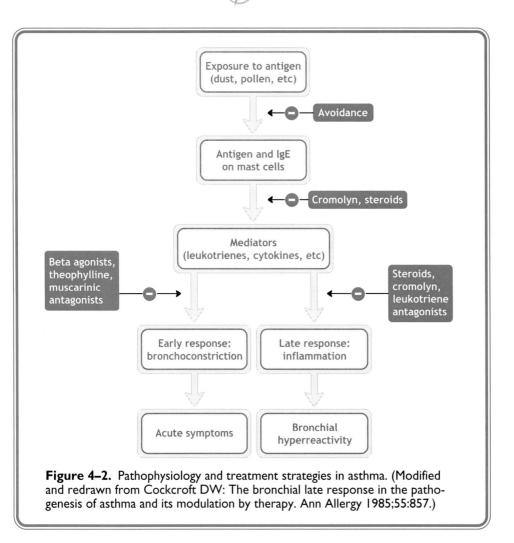

Figure 4–2. Pathophysiology and treatment strategies in asthma. (Modified and redrawn from Cockcroft DW: The bronchial late response in the pathogenesis of asthma and its modulation by therapy. Ann Allergy 1985;55:857.)

    b. Toxicity consists of dry mouth and, rarely, tachycardia and cycloplegia.

   3. Theophylline is a methylxanthine related to caffeine and theobromine, but is a more effective bronchodilator than either.

    a. It acts by inhibiting phosphodiesterase, an enzyme that breaks down cAMP.

    b. It is not active by the inhaled route and the drug is usually used orally.

    c. Systemic toxicities (GI disturbances, tremor, arrhythmias, and convulsions in overdose) are possible.

 C. The anti-inflammatory drugs used in asthma include **corticosteroids, mast cell stabilizers,** and **leukotriene antagonists.**

   1. Corticosteroids are the most important prophylactic agents for asthma and are given by metered-dose inhaler whenever possible to minimize systemic toxicity.

    a. Steroids commonly used in asthma include **beclomethasone, fluticasone,** and several others.

b. These drugs act by inhibiting the production and release of leukotrienes and inflammatory cytokines.

    c. When inhalational therapy is not adequate, oral or even parenteral administration is used to control airway inflammation and symptoms.

    d. Toxicities of inhaled corticosteroids include temporary retardation of growth in young children and candidal yeast infection of the larynx. Toxicities of systemic corticosteroids are described in Chapter 6.

2. Mast cell stabilizers include **cromolyn** and **nedocromil,** highly insoluble compounds that can be administered by metered-dose inhaler with practically no absorption or systemic toxicity.

    a. These drugs probably act by inhibiting mast cell release of inflammatory and allergic mediators, including leukotrienes, cytokines, and histamine.

    b. Cromolyn is also available in formulations for the treatment of ocular, nasal, and gastrointestinal allergic conditions.

3. Leukotriene receptor antagonists include **zafirlukast** and **montelukast.**

    a. These drugs are orally active, an advantage for treatment of young children and others who cannot use inhalers.

    b. They are not as effective as corticosteroids and have no value in acute bronchospasm.

CLINICAL PROBLEMS

A 26-year-old woman comes to an allergy clinic complaining of a runny nose and itching eyes. The symptoms become particularly severe during the spring months. She has tried over-the-counter antihistamines and they help reduce the symptoms, but also cause side effects that she finds intolerable.

1. Which of the following drugs would you **not** recommend?

    A. Cetirizine

    B. Desloratadine

    C. Diphenhydramine

    D. Fexofenadine

    E. Loratadine

A 45-year-old man is to undergo chemotherapy for a testicular tumor.

2. Which of the following drugs is most likely to be used concomitantly as an antiemetic?

    A. Bromocriptine

    B. Ergotamine

    C. Ibuprofen

    D. Ondansetron

    E. Sumatriptan

A 63-year-old man has glaucoma and requires treatment to lower the intraocular pressure.

3. Which of the following eicosanoids is most likely to be used?

   A. Alprostadil

   B. Dinoprostone

   C. Latanoprost

   D. Misoprostol

   E. Prostacyclin

A 65-year-old woman comes to your office with a complaint of black stools and "feeling weak." Stool testing for occult blood is strongly positive and her hemoglobin is 8 g/dL (normal 12–14 g/dL). Medical history reveals that she has had rheumatoid arthritis for 15 years. On a doctor's recommendation, she has treated her symptoms with aspirin with good control of her symptoms. Your diagnosis is gastrointestinal bleeding due to the NSAID.

4. Which of the following drugs will control her rheumatoid arthritis symptoms with the smallest risk of bleeding?

   A. Diclofenac

   B. Ibuprofen

   C. Ketorolac

   D. Naproxen

   E. Valdecoxib

A 57-year-old man has been found in a screening program to have elevated total cholesterol (285 mg/dL, desirable <200 mg/dL) and elevated triglycerides. He has a family history of early cardiovascular disease.

5. Which of the following drugs should **not** be used in his treatment?

   A. Atorvastatin

   B. Colestipol

   C. Gemfibrozil

   D. Lovastatin

   E. Niacin

ANSWERS

1. The answer is C. All of the drugs listed are second-generation, nonsedating antihistamines except diphenhydramine. Diphenhydramine is strongly sedating and has significant autonomic blocking actions.

2. The answer is D. Ondansetron, a 5-HT$_3$ antagonist, is an effective antiemetic agent and is heavily used in chemotherapy and following general anesthesia. The other drugs listed do not have antiemetic action.

3. The answer is C. Latanoprost, a $PGF_{2\alpha}$ analog, is a useful topical antiglaucoma therapy. It probably acts by increasing aqueous outflow.

4. The answer is E. All of the drugs listed are effective NSAIDs and are capable of reducing symptoms of rheumatoid arthritis. However, all except valdecoxib are relatively nonselective inhibitors of COX-1 and COX-2, and are therefore likely to cause GI bleeding. Valdecoxib (and celecoxib) are selective COX-2 inhibitors and reduce inflammation with a lower risk of GI bleeding, although they carry a higher risk of cardiovascular toxicity.

5. The answer is B. The bile acid–binding resins, colestipol and cholestyramine, are often associated with increases in VLDL and triglycerides. They should not be used in patients with significant hypertriglyceridemia. Niacin and the fibrates are primary agents for triglyceridemia. Atorvastatin is the statin most effective in lowering triglycerides as well as LDL levels.

CHAPTER 5
CENTRAL NERVOUS SYSTEM DRUGS

I. Introduction to Central Nervous System (CNS) Drugs

A. Targets of CNS Drug Action

1. **Voltage-regulated ion channels** include Na^+ channels in axonal membranes and Ca^{2+} channels in presynaptic membranes.

2. **Neurotransmitter-regulated ion channels** are of two main types.

   a. Directly coupled (no second messenger) ion channels include the Cl^- channel regulated by γ-aminobutyric acid ($GABA_A$) receptors.

   b. G protein coupled ion channels [using cyclic AMP (cAMP), inositol trisphosphate (IP_3), and diacylglycerol (DAG) as second messengers] include most CNS neurotransmitter systems.

B. CNS Transmitters

1. Major CNS neurotransmitters include glutamic acid, GABA, acetylcholine, dopamine, norepinephrine, serotonin, and the opioid peptides.

2. These CNS neurotransmitters, including their receptors and drug actions, are listed in Table 5–1.

C. Sites of CNS Drug Actions

1. The effects of most therapeutically important CNS drugs are exerted mainly at synapses.

2. Possible mechanisms of CNS drugs are illustrated in Figure 5–1.

II. Sedative-Hypnotics

A. Classification & Pharmacokinetics

1. Subclasses of **sedative-hypnotics** include **benzodiazepines** (Table 5–2), **carbamates** (meprobamate), **barbiturates** (phenobarbital and secobarbital), **alcohols** (ethanol and chloral hydrate), newer drugs (zolpidem and zaleplon), and the selective anxiolytic buspirone.

2. Sedative-hypnotics are metabolized by hepatic enzymes, with some forming active metabolites (eg, diazepam and chloral hydrate). The duration of effects varies from a few hours (eg, triazolam and zolpidem) to more than a day (eg, diazepam and phenobarbital).

B. Mechanisms of Action

1. **Benzodiazepines** (BZs) bind to components (BZ receptors) of the $GABA_A$ receptor–chloride ion channel macromolecular complex (Figure 5–2), increasing the inhibitory actions of GABA. This action is reversed by the BZ receptor antagonist flumazenil.

Table 5–1. CNS neurotransmitters.

Transmitter	Receptors	Drug Actions
Glutamic acid	Excitatory	Antagonized by ketamine, phencyclidine, and newer antiepileptics
GABA	Inhibitory	Sedative-hypnotics and antiepileptic drugs facilitate $GABA_A$ receptors; baclofen activates $GABA_B$ receptors
Acetylcholine	M_1, excitatory; M_2, inhibitory; N, excitatory	M blockers (eg, atropine) antagonize both M_1 and M_2 receptors; AChE inhibitors facilitate ACh
Dopamine	Inhibitory	Antagonized by older antipsychotics; activated by anti-parkinsonian drugs, amphetamines, and cocaine
Norepinephrine	Excitatory or inhibitory	Amplified by MAO inhibitors, tricyclic antidepressants, amphetamines, and cocaine
Serotonin	Excitatory or inhibitory	Amplified by MAO inhibitors, selective serotonin reuptake inhibitors, tricyclic antidepressants, some CNS stimulants, and hallucinogens
Opioid peptides	Inhibitory	Amplified by opioid analgesics; antagonized by naloxone and naltrexone

2. **Barbiturates** facilitate GABA actions via binding to a separate site from the BZ receptors; their actions are not reversed by flumazenil. Barbiturates also antagonize glutamate receptors and block Na^+ channels.
3. **Zolpidem** and zaleplon act via BZ receptors; their actions are reversed by flumazenil.
4. **Alcohols** may facilitate GABA (not via BZ receptors) or block glutamate receptors.

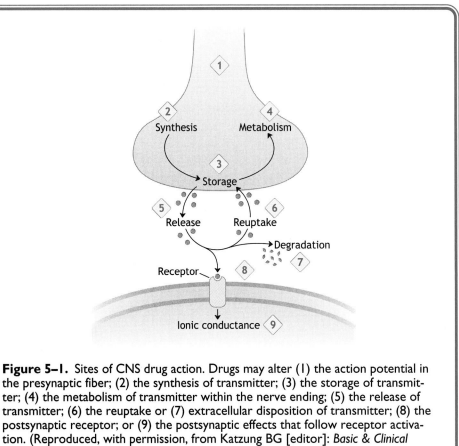

Figure 5–1. Sites of CNS drug action. Drugs may alter (1) the action potential in the presynaptic fiber; (2) the synthesis of transmitter; (3) the storage of transmitter; (4) the metabolism of transmitter within the nerve ending; (5) the release of transmitter; (6) the reuptake or (7) extracellular disposition of transmitter; (8) the postsynaptic receptor; or (9) the postsynaptic effects that follow receptor activation. (Reproduced, with permission, from Katzung BG [editor]: *Basic & Clinical Pharmacology,* 9th ed. McGraw-Hill, 2004.)

  5. **Buspirone** is a partial agonist at 5-hydroxytryptamine (5-HT$_{1A}$) receptors; its anxiolytic onset may take 1–2 weeks.

C. **Pharmacodynamics**
  1. Dose-dependent CNS depression includes sedation, hypnosis, anesthesia, and coma.
  2. Most sedative-hypnotics suppress rapid eye movement (REM) sleep and REM "rebound" may occur on abrupt discontinuance.
  3. Benzodiazepines cause anterograde amnesia and exert both muscle-relaxing and anticonvulsant actions.
  4. Tolerance and dependence develop with chronic use. Abrupt discontinuance may result in an abstinence or withdrawal syndrome characterized by agitation, tremors, hyperreflexia, and seizures. This syndrome does not occur on discontinuance of buspirone.

D. **Clinical Uses**
  1. Sedative-hypnotics are used to treat generalized anxiety states, panic attacks, phobic disorders, sleep disorders, muscle spasticity states, and seizure disorders.

Table 5–2. Characteristics of selected sedative-hypnotics.

Drug	Indications	Specific Characteristics
Alprazolam	Anxiety, panic attacks, phobias	
Diazepam	Anxiety, preoperative sedation, muscle relaxation, withdrawal states, status epilepticus	Long-acting BZ
Midazolam	Preoperative sedation, intravenous anesthesia	Shortest-acting BZ
Triazolam	Sleep disorders	Short-acting BZ
Phenobarbital	Anxiety, seizures, withdrawal states	Very long-acting
Secobarbital	Sleep disorders	Short-acting; high abuse potential
Zolpidem	Sleep disorders	Minimal daytime sedation
Buspirone	Generalized anxiety	Not a CNS depressant; slow onset; no abuse liability

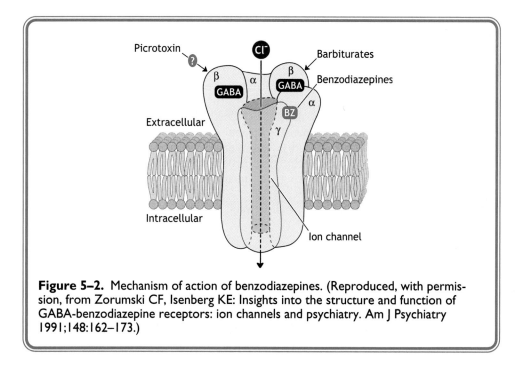

Figure 5–2. Mechanism of action of benzodiazepines. (Reproduced, with permission, from Zorumski CF, Isenberg KE: Insights into the structure and function of GABA-benzodiazepine receptors: ion channels and psychiatry. Am J Psychiatry 1991;148:162–173.)

      2. Longer-acting drugs (eg, diazepam) with dose tapering are used to suppress withdrawal symptoms.

    E. Toxicities

      1. Pharmacodynamic actions include CNS depression, resulting in cognitive impairment, unwanted daytime sedation, and decreased psychomotor skills. Overdose causes depression of respiratory and vasomotor drive.

      2. Drug interactions include additive CNS depression. Barbiturates induce liver drug-metabolizing enzymes and also precipitate acute porphyric attacks. Chloral hydrate displaces warfarin from plasma proteins.

DRUG TREATMENT OF ANXIETY STATES AND SLEEP DISORDERS

CLINICAL CORRELATION

- *In addition to benzodiazepines, drugs useful in panic attacks and phobic disorders include tricyclic antidepressants (eg, imipramine), monoamine oxidase (MAO) inhibitors (eg, phenelzine), and selective serotonin reuptake inhibitors (SSRIs).*
- *Generalized anxiety disorders respond to buspirone and SSRIs (eg, paroxetine) as well as to benzodiazepines.*
- *Zolpidem, zaleplon, and triazolam are commonly used in sleep disorders.*
- *Shorter-acting barbiturates, chloral hydrate, and drugs other than sedative-hypnotics (eg, promethazine) can also be used as "sleeping pills."*

    F. Ethanol

      1. Ethanol is initially metabolized via **alcohol dehydrogenase (ADH)** (Figure 5–3).

        a. The high affinity of ethanol for ADH is used competitively in methanol and ethylene glycol poisoning to prevent formation of toxic metabolites.

        b. Fomepizole, an ADH inhibitor, is also used for this purpose.

        c. Acetaldehyde formed from ethanol is metabolized to acetate via aldehyde dehydrogenase, an enzyme inhibited by disulfiram and other drugs.

      2. Initial effects include dose-dependent sedation, impaired judgment, slurred speech, ataxia, and coma.

        a. Ethanol is a vasodilator and is cardiodepressant.

        b. Management of acute toxicity includes ventilatory support, dextrose, and thiamine.

      3. Chronic effects include tolerance and dependence (withdrawal symptoms may be severe and include delirium tremens), gastrointestinal (GI) irritation, hepatic dysfunction, peripheral neuropathy, the Wernicke-Korsakoff syndrome (thiamine deficiency), and endocrine dysfunction. Ethanol is teratogenic (fetal alcohol syndrome) resulting in mental retardation and craniofacial abnormalities.

      4. Treatment of alcoholism may involve use of disulfiram, naltrexone, and antidepressants.

  III. Antiepileptic Drugs (AEDs)

    A. The mechanisms of action of AEDs are given in Table 5–3.

    B. The characteristics of conventional AEDs are given in Table 5–4.

    C. Clinical uses depend on specific seizure type.

      1. Generalized tonic–clonic and partial seizures are treated with phenytoin, carbamazepine, or valproic acid.

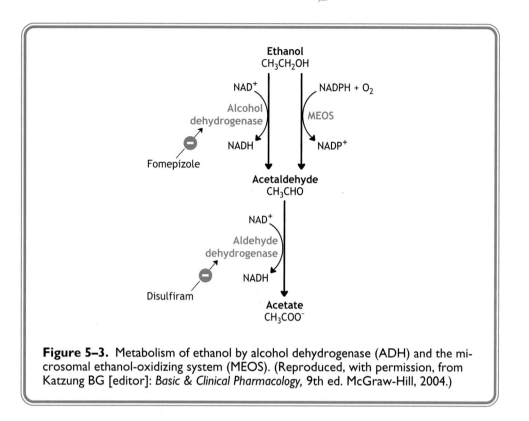

Figure 5–3. Metabolism of ethanol by alcohol dehydrogenase (ADH) and the microsomal ethanol-oxidizing system (MEOS). (Reproduced, with permission, from Katzung BG [editor]: *Basic & Clinical Pharmacology*, 9th ed. McGraw-Hill, 2004.)

    2. Absence seizures are treated with ethosuximide or valproic acid.
    3. Myoclonic syndromes are treated with valproic acid.
    4. Status epilepticus is treated with intravenous diazepam, lorazepam, phenytoin, or phenobarbital.
  D. Toxicities of conventional AEDs are given in Table 5–4.
  E. Characteristics of newer AEDs are given in Table 5–5.

Table 5–3. Mechanisms of action of antiepileptic drugs.

Mechanism of Action	Drugs
GABA potentiation	Benzodiazepines, barbiturates, gabapentin, tiagabine, and vigabatrin
Na^+ ion channel block	Carbamazepine and phenytoin; high doses of barbiturates and valproic acid
Ca^{2+} ion channel block	Ethosuximide and valproic acid
Glutamic acid antagonism	Felbamate, lamotrigine, and topiramate

Table 5–4. Characteristics of older antiepileptic drugs.

Drug	Characteristic Features	Toxicities
Carbamazepine	Used in partial and tonic–clonic seizures; also used in trigeminal neuralgia and bipolar disorders	CNS depression, hematotoxicity, induces drug-metabolizing enzymes,[1] teratogenic (craniofacial anomalies)
Clonazepam	Used in myoclonic seizures; also used in anxiety states, migraine, and bipolar disorders	Sedation is dose-limiting; dependence liability
Ethosuximide	Only used in absence seizures	Gastrointestinal distress, lethargy, headache
Phenobarbital	Back-up drug in tonic–clonic and partial seizures; also used in anxiety and withdrawal states	CNS depression, dependence liability, induces drug-metabolizing enzymes[1]
Phenytoin	Used in partial and tonic–clonic seizures; also used in bipolar disorder; pharmacokinetic features include variable oral absorption, competition for plasma protein binding, and induction of drug-metabolizing enzymes[1]	CNS depression, hematotoxicity, hirsutism, gingival hyperplasia, osteomalacia, teratogenic (craniofacial anomalies)
Valproic acid	"Broadest spectrum" AED used in absence, myoclonic, partial, and tonic–clonic seizures; also used in bipolar disorder and migraine	Gastrointestinal distress hepatotoxicity, inhibition of drug metabolism, teratogenic (spina bifida)

[1]AEDs may decrease the efficacy of oral contraceptives.

ORAL CONTRACEPTIVES IN EPILEPSY

- Antiepileptic drugs that induce drug-metabolizing enzymes may enhance the metabolism of estrogenic steroids, possibly decreasing the effectiveness of oral contraceptives.
- Patients treated with such drugs, including carbamazepine, phenobarbital, and phenytoin, are advised to consider alternative contraceptive methods to avoid pregnancy.
- This is especially important given the teratogenic potential of many antiepileptic drugs.

Table 5–5. Characteristics of newer antiepileptic drugs.

Drug	Clinical Uses	Toxicities
Felbamate	Back-up in partial seizures, Lennox-Gastaut syndrome, and myoclonic syndromes	Aplastic anemia, hepato-toxicity
Gabapentin	Partial seizures, bipolar disorder, neuropathic pain, migraine	Sedation, movement disorders, leukopenia
Lamotrigine	Back-up in absence and partial seizures	Sedation, hematotoxicity, skin reactions (life-threatening)
Tiagabine	Back-up in partial seizures	Dizziness, tremor
Topiramate	Back-up in partial seizures	Sedation, emotional lability, tremor, weight loss
Vigabatrin	Back-up in partial seizures	Sedation, weight gain, confusion, ocular toxicity

IV. General Anesthetics

A. Concepts

1. General anesthesia includes unconsciousness, analgesia, amnesia, muscle relaxation, and loss of reflexes.
2. Anesthesia protocols involve use of **inhaled** and/or **intravenous anesthetics,** often with skeletal muscle relaxants and local anesthetics.

B. Inhaled Anesthetics

1. Agents include nitrous oxide and halogenated hydrocarbons (Table 5–6).
2. Mechanisms of action include blockade of membrane Na^+ channels and/or activation of GABA-mediated Cl^- ion flux.
3. **MAC value** (minimal alveolar anesthetic concentration, as percentage of inspired air) is inversely related to anesthetic gas potency. MAC values are used in calculating dosage, are additive, and decrease with increasing age of the patient.
4. **Blood:gas solubility ratio** of inhaled agents determines both rate of onset and recovery. Agents with low ratios (eg, nitrous oxide and desflurane) have an onset more rapid and a duration of anesthesia shorter than agents with high blood solubility (eg, enflurane and halothane).
5. Pharmacodynamic actions include increased cerebral blood flow, uterine smooth muscle relaxation, and decreased ventilatory response to hypoxia.

C. Intravenous Anesthetics

1. **Thiopental,** a barbiturate, has a rapid onset (anesthesia induction) and short duration due to redistribution from brain to other tissues. It decreases cerebral blood flow.

Table 5–6. Characteristics of inhaled anesthetics.

Agent	MAC Value (% of inspired air)	Blood: Gas Solubility Ratio	CV Effects	Specific Characteristics
Nitrous oxide	>100	0.47	Minimal	Low potency; rapid onset and recovery
Desflurane	6.5	0.42	Vasodilation	Airway irritation; rapid recovery
Sevoflurane	2.0	0.69	Myocardial depression	Rapid onset and recovery
Enflurane	1.7	1.8	Myocardial depression	Tonic–clonic muscle spasms
Isoflurane	1.4	1.4	Vasodilation	Bronchiolar secretion and spasms
Halothane	0.8	2.3	Myocardial depression	Hepatitis; sensitizes myocardium to endogenous amines

2. **Midazolam** is a benzodiazepine with amnestic effects. Recovery can be facilitated by flumazenil.
3. **Fentanyl** and related opioids have fewer cardiovascular actions than inhaled anesthetics. Recovery can be facilitated by naloxone.
4. **Propofol** has a rapid onset, fast recovery, and antiemetic actions.
5. **Ketamine** causes "dissociative anesthesia," with emergence reactions, and cardiovascular stimulation.

V. Local Anesthetics
   A. Pharmacokinetics
     1. **Disposition:** Esters (eg, procaine) are usually inactivated by plasma cholinesterases; amides (eg, lidocaine and bupivacaine) are inactivated by liver enzymes.
     2. **Systemic absorption:** With the exception of cocaine, local anesthetics are rapidly absorbed into the blood; coadministration of an α agonist prolongs action.
   B. Mechanism of Action
     1. **Ionization:** Local anesthetics cross membranes in their nonionized form, but their ionized forms interact with components of the Na^+ channel located on the inside of excitable membranes (Figure 5–4).

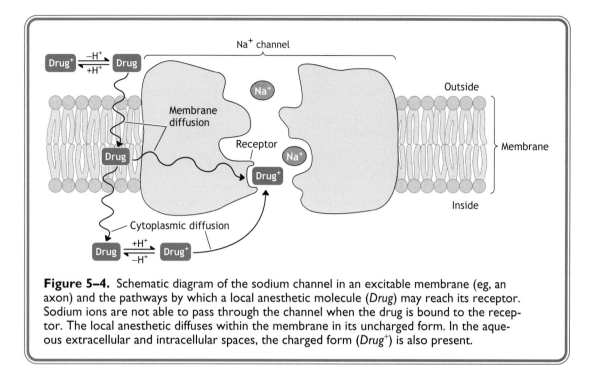

Figure 5–4. Schematic diagram of the sodium channel in an excitable membrane (eg, an axon) and the pathways by which a local anesthetic molecule (*Drug*) may reach its receptor. Sodium ions are not able to pass through the channel when the drug is bound to the receptor. The local anesthetic diffuses within the membrane in its uncharged form. In the aqueous extracellular and intracellular spaces, the charged form (*Drug⁺*) is also present.

      2. State-dependent action: Local anesthetics interact with Na⁺ channels in their open or inactivated states. Small-diameter, rapidly firing fibers (including type A_δ and type C fibers) are most sensitive.

  C. Toxicities

      1. CNS effects can vary from sedation to seizures.

      2. Cardiovascular effects include vasodilation and myocardial depression (except for cocaine).

      3. Allergic reactions have occurred with local anesthetic esters via *para*-aminobenzoic acid (PABA) formation.

VI. Skeletal Muscle Relaxants

  A. Concepts

      1. Neuromuscular (NM) blockers are used to provide muscle paralysis to facilitate surgery or assisted ventilation.

      2. Spasmolytic drugs reduce abnormally elevated tone caused by neurologic dysfunction or muscle disease.

  B. Nondepolarizing NM Blockers

      1. Tubocurarine is the prototype; related drugs vary in their pharmacokinetic and pharmacodynamic properties (Table 5–7).

      2. Mechanism of action: Competitive antagonism prevents depolarization by acetylcholine (ACh) at the skeletal muscle end plate (Figure 5–5). This is reversible by acetylcholinesterase (AChE) inhibitors.

      3. Toxicities include respiratory paralysis and autonomic effects.

Table 5–7. Characteristics of neuromuscular blockers.

Drug	Pharmacokinetics	Pharmacodynamics
Tubocurarine	Renal elimination; long duration of action	Blocks ANS ganglia; causes histamine release
Atracurium	Spontaneous breakdown	Minimal ANS effects
Mivacurium	Metabolized by plasma cholinesterase; short action	Minimal ANS effects
Pancuronium	Renal elimination; long action	Blocks cardiac muscarinic receptors
Vecuronium	Biliary elimination; short duration	No ANS effects
Succinylcholine	Metabolized by plasma cholinesterase	Stimulates ANS ganglia and cardiac muscarinic receptor

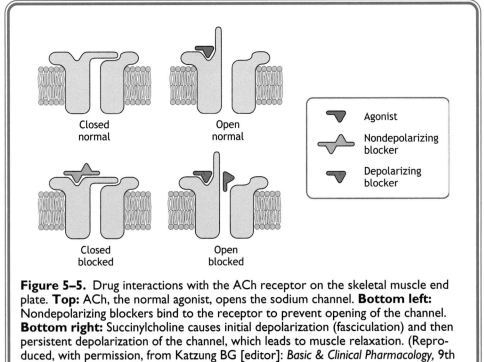

Closed normal

Open normal

Closed blocked

Open blocked

▼ Agonist

▲▼▲ Nondepolarizing blocker

▼ Depolarizing blocker

Figure 5–5. Drug interactions with the ACh receptor on the skeletal muscle end plate. **Top:** ACh, the normal agonist, opens the sodium channel. **Bottom left:** Nondepolarizing blockers bind to the receptor to prevent opening of the channel. **Bottom right:** Succinylcholine causes initial depolarization (fasciculation) and then persistent depolarization of the channel, which leads to muscle relaxation. (Reproduced, with permission, from Katzung BG [editor]: *Basic & Clinical Pharmacology,* 9th ed. McGraw-Hill, 2004.)

C. **Depolarizing NM Blocker**
1. **Succinylcholine** has a short duration of action (3–6 minutes) following a single dose due to rapid metabolism via plasma cholinesterases; some patients experience prolonged duration of action due to enzyme deficiency (genotypic variation).
2. **Mechanism of action:** The end plate is depolarized causing brief fasciculations followed by a flaccid paralysis (phase I), which is not reversed by AChE inhibitors. With continuous infusion the muscle end plate repolarizes (phase II) but remains blocked (similar to nondepolarizing blockade).
3. **Toxicities** include GI distress, emesis, muscle pain, and hyperkalemia.

D. **Spasmolytics**
1. **Diazepam** facilitates $GABA_A$-mediated presynaptic inhibition.
2. **Baclofen** activates $GABA_B$ receptors in the spinal cord.
3. **Dantrolene** decreases Ca^{2+} release from the sarcoplasmic reticulum in skeletal muscle, but causes significant weakness.
4. **Cyclobenzaprine** acts centrally to decrease an acute spasm due to muscle injury, but is ineffective in cerebral palsy or spinal cord injury.

MALIGNANT HYPERTHERMIA

- *Anesthesia protocols that use halogenated inhalational agents together with muscle relaxants such as tubocurarine and succinylcholine may cause malignant hyperthermia.*
- *This is a rare life-threatening condition with muscle rigidity, autonomic lability, and seizures, due to uncontrolled release of Ca^{2+} from the sarcoplasmic reticulum.*
- *Variations in the ryanodine receptor gene may be responsible for its occurrence in some patients.*
- *Dantrolene, which blocks calcium release, is used to manage the symptoms of malignant hyperthermia.*

VII. Drugs for Parkinsonism and Other Movement Disorders

A. **Concepts**
1. **Parkinson's disease** involves loss of dopaminergic activity in the striatum, resulting in excessive actions of ACh (Figure 5–6).
   a. Drugs that enhance dopaminergic activity or decrease cholinergic activity are used.
   b. Reversible extrapyramidal dysfunction with symptoms resembling parkinsonism is caused by antipsychotic drugs that block striatal dopamine receptors.
2. In **Huntington's disease** GABA functions are decreased and dopaminergic functions are enhanced (Figure 5–6). Drugs that block dopamine receptors are ameliorative.

B. **Levodopa**
1. **Mechanism of action:** Levodopa is actively accumulated in the CNS where it is converted by dopa decarboxylase to dopamine; it is used with carbidopa, an inhibitor of peripheral decarboxylase.
2. **Clinical use:** Levodopa is widely used in parkinsonism.
3. **Toxicities** include dyskinesias, hypotension, gastrointestinal distress, behavioral effects, and rapid fluctuations in clinical response (the "on-off" phenomenon).

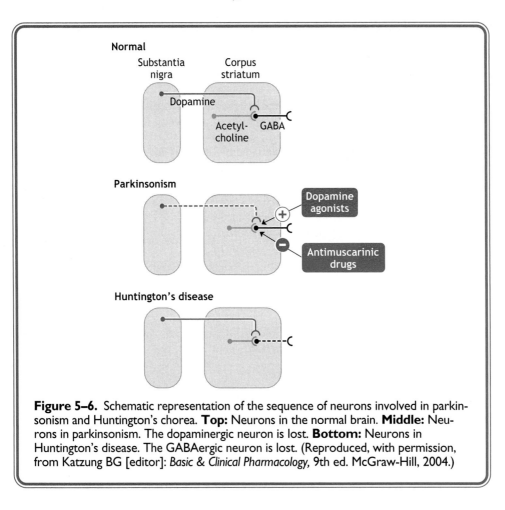

Figure 5–6. Schematic representation of the sequence of neurons involved in parkinsonism and Huntington's chorea. **Top:** Neurons in the normal brain. **Middle:** Neurons in parkinsonism. The dopaminergic neuron is lost. **Bottom:** Neurons in Huntington's disease. The GABAergic neuron is lost. (Reproduced, with permission, from Katzung BG [editor]: *Basic & Clinical Pharmacology,* 9th ed. McGraw-Hill, 2004.)

    C. **Bromocriptine and Pergolide**
        1. **Mechanism and use:** These ergot derivatives activate striatal dopamine (DA) receptors; they are used as individual agents or in drug combinations.
        2. **Toxicities** include gastrointestinal effects, dyskinesias, hypotension, hallucinations, pulmonary infiltrates, and erythromelalgia.
    D. **Pramipexole and Ropinirole**
        1. **Mechanism and use:** These drugs activate striatal DA receptors; they are first-line drugs in early treatment.
        2. **Toxicities** include dyskinesias, hypotension, lassitude, and sleepiness.
    E. **Antimuscarinics**
        1. **Mechanism of action:** Benztropine and similar drugs block striatal muscarinic receptors.
        2. **Clinical uses:** These drugs are adjunctive in parkinsonism, improving tremor and rigidity, but not motility. They alleviate reversible extrapyramidal effects caused by older antipsychotic drugs.
        3. **Toxicities** include drowsiness, confusion, and delusions; peripheral effects are atropinelike.

F. Other Agents Used in Parkinsonism
1. **Selegiline** inhibits MAO type B, which metabolizes dopamine.
   a. It is used adjunctively and as the sole agent in early treatment.
   b. Hepatic metabolism results in the formation of amphetamine.
   c. Toxicities include insomnia, dyskinesias, and hypotension.
2. **Entacapone** and **tolcapone** are **catechol-*O*-methyltransferase (COMT) inhibitors.**
   a. They block conversion of levodopa to 3-*O*-methyldopa, which may compete with levodopa for uptake into the CNS.
   b. These drugs are used adjunctively with levodopa to improve responsivity.
   c. Tolcapone is hepatotoxic.
3. **Amantadine** enhances dopaminergic functions and/or blocks muscarinic receptors. Toxicities include behavioral effects and dermatotoxicity.

EFFICACY OF LEVODOPA IN PARKINSON'S DISEASE

- *In most patients the effectiveness of levodopa begins to decline after 5 years of treatment.*
- *There are two likely explanations for this loss of therapeutic activity.*
  - *The first is progressive degeneration of nigrostriatal neurons to the point that few nerve endings are available for the conversion of levodopa to dopamine.*
  - *The second is neurotoxicity due to levodopa-induced oxidative stress.*

G. Drugs for Other Movement Disorders
1. **Huntington's disease** is treated with **haloperidol** and **phenothiazines,** which block dopamine receptors, or **tetrabenazine,** which depletes brain amines.
2. **Tourette's syndrome** is treated with **haloperidol** and **pimozide.**
3. **Drug-induced dyskinesias** are treated with **muscarinic blockers,** which ameliorate reversible extrapyramidal dysfunction.
4. **Tremor** is treated with **propranolol.**
5. **Wilson's disease** is treated with **penicillamine.**

VIII. Drugs for Psychoses and Bipolar Disorder

A. Concepts
1. The **dopamine hypothesis** proposes that schizophrenia may result from a "functional excess" of dopamine in the CNS. Drugs that block dopamine receptors can ameliorate schizophrenic symptoms; drugs that activate dopamine receptors exacerbate symptoms or cause psychoses.
2. Efficacy of older antipsychotic drugs correlates with their affinity as antagonists for brain dopamine D_2 receptors. Blockade of this receptor in the striatum results in extrapyramidal dysfunction.
3. Newer antipsychotic drugs have low affinity for D_2 receptors and high affinity for serotonin 5-HT_{2A} receptors. Extrapyramidal dysfunction is reduced and negative symptoms of schizophrenia may improve.

B. Antipsychotic Agents
1. **Classification:** Older antipsychotic drugs include phenothiazines (eg, **chlorpromazine, thioridazine,** and **trifluoperazine**) and butyrophenones (eg, **haloperidol**). Newer antipsychotic drugs include **clozapine, olanzapine, risperidone, quetiapine, ziprasidone,** and **aripiprazole.**
2. **Pharmacokinetics:** These well-absorbed drugs sequester in body tissues (long half-lives) and require metabolism for elimination.

C. **Pharmacodynamics**
1. **Dopamine receptor antagonism** is the basis for the antipsychotic actions of older drugs and their efficacy as antiemetics and is responsible for extrapyramidal dysfunction and hyperprolactinemia.
2. **Muscarinic receptor antagonism** causes atropinelike side effects, especially with thioridazine and clozapine.
3. **α-Adrenoceptor antagonism** causes the hypotensive actions of phenothiazines and clozapine.
4. **Histamine H_1 receptor antagonism** is the basis for use of some phenothiazines as antihistaminics.
5. **Sedation** is marked with phenothiazines.

D. **Clinical Uses**
1. Antipsychotic drugs reduce the positive symptoms of **schizophrenia** and facilitate patient functionality; they have a slow onset (weeks).
2. Other uses include initial treatment of mania, maintenance in bipolar disorders (newer drugs), schizoaffective disorders, Tourette's syndrome (haloperidol and molindone), Huntington's chorea (haloperidol), drug-induced toxic psychosis, and possibly psychiatric symptoms associated with Alzheimer's disease and parkinsonism (newer agents). Phenothiazines (eg, prochlorperazine) are used as antiemetics.

E. **Toxicities**
1. **Extrapyramidal dysfunction:** Reversible effects include parkinsonian symptoms, akathisias, and acute dystonias. Management includes lowering the dose, using muscarinic receptor antagonists, or changing to a newer antipsychotic drug.
2. **Tardive dyskinesias:** Late-occurring, choreoathetoid-like movements are caused mainly by older drugs and may be irreversible.
   a. They are possibly due to dopamine receptor supersensitivity.
   b. There is no antidote but symptoms may respond to tetrabenazine.
   c. Clozapine does not exacerbate the symptoms.
3. **Endocrine and metabolic effects:** Amenorrhea-galactorrhea and gynecomastia are caused by older drugs. Newer drugs may cause metabolic dysfunction including weight gain and disorders of carbohydrate metabolism.
4. **Neuroleptic malignant syndrome:** This is a rare syndrome similar to malignant hyperthermia.
5. **Overdose toxicity:** Symptoms result from receptor blocking actions and CNS depression; most drugs lower the seizure threshold.
6. **Specific toxicities** include agranulocytosis (clozapine) and cardiotoxicity and retinal pigmentation (thioridazine).

NEUROCHEMICAL IMBALANCE IN THE CNS

CLINICAL CORRELATION

- *In Parkinson's disease the loss of nigrostriatal dopaminergic neurons leads to excessive cholinergic activity with resulting extrapyramidal dysfunction; dopaminergic agonists or muscarinic blockers or both are used in treatment.*
- *In schizophrenia, excessive dopaminergic activity may be attenuated by drugs that block dopamine receptors; in Huntington's chorea, symptoms may be alleviated by dopamine receptor–blocking agents.*
- *In major depression pharmacologic management involves drugs that may rectify a "functional deficiency" in noradrenergic or serotonergic neurotransmission.*

F. **Lithium and Other Drugs for Bipolar Disorder**

1. **Pharmacokinetics:** Lithium is well absorbed orally, distributes in total body water, and undergoes renal elimination. Due to a narrow therapeutic window, plasma levels should be monitored initially.

2. **Mechanism of action:** Lithium inhibits recycling of membrane phosphatidylinositol bisphosphate (PIP_2) by blocking dephosphorylation of inositol diphosphate.

3. **Clinical use:** Lithium is the standard drug for maintenance in bipolar disorder.

4. **Toxicities:** Adverse neurologic effects include tremor, sedation, aphasia, and ataxia. Lithium may cause acne, edema, goiter, and diabetes insipidus. It is teratogenic (cardiac malformations).

5. **Alternative drugs:** Carbamazepine, clonazepam, gabapentin, lamotrigine, valproic acid, and olanzapine are all effective.

IX. **Antidepressants**

A. **Concepts**

1. The **amine hypothesis of depression** posits that a functional decrease in brain norepinephrine and/or serotonin is responsible for the disorder.

2. Most drugs effective in major depression appear to facilitate the activity of brain amines.

B. **Drug Classes & Actions on CNS Amines**

1. **Monoamine oxidase inhibitors** (**MAOIs**) (eg, **phenelzine**) inhibit MAO type A, which results in an increase in presynaptic levels of norepinephrine and serotonin.

2. **Tricyclics** (**TCAs**) (eg, **amitriptyline, imipramine,** and **clomipramine**) block neuronal reuptake of norepinephrine and serotonin, increasing their postsynaptic actions.

3. **Selective serotonin reuptake inhibitors** (**SSRIs**) (eg, **fluoxetine, citalopram, paroxetine,** and **sertraline**) block neuronal reuptake of serotonin.

4. **Heterocyclic second- and third-generation antidepressants** have varied actions (Figure 5–7).

   a. **Amoxapine** and **maprotiline** block norepinephrine reuptake.

   b. **Mirtazapine** antagonizes presynaptic α_2 receptors, increasing norepinephrine release.

   c. **Trazodone** blocks serotonin reuptake.

   d. **Venlafaxine** blocks reuptake of norepinephrine and serotonin.

   e. **Bupropion** has no significant action on norepinephrine or serotonin.

C. **Pharmacodynamics**

1. **CNS actions:** In addition to the effects on brain amines, TCAs and most heterocyclics (especially mirtazapine and trazodone) cause sedation, additive with other CNS depressants. SSRIs, bupropion, and venlafaxine may cause anxiety, insomnia, and jitteriness. Most of these drugs cause seizures in overdose.

2. **Peripheral actions:** TCAs, amoxapine, maprotiline, and nefazodone cause atropinelike side effects via muscarinic receptor antagonism.

   a. Weight gain occurs with TCAs and MAOIs; weight loss is common with SSRIs.

   b. Drug interactions may occur via inhibition of hepatic cytochrome P-450 isoenzymes by nefazodone, SSRIs, and venlafaxine.

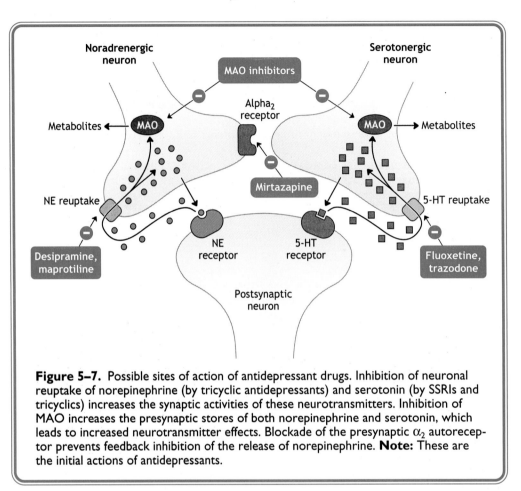

Figure 5–7. Possible sites of action of antidepressant drugs. Inhibition of neuronal reuptake of norepinephrine (by tricyclic antidepressants) and serotonin (by SSRIs and tricyclics) increases the synaptic activities of these neurotransmitters. Inhibition of MAO increases the presynaptic stores of both norepinephrine and serotonin, which leads to increased neurotransmitter effects. Blockade of the presynaptic α_2 autoreceptor prevents feedback inhibition of the release of norepinephrine. **Note:** These are the initial actions of antidepressants.

    c. MAOIs also inhibit metabolism of certain sympathomimetic amines and tyramine with potential for hypertensive reactions.

D. Clinical Uses

   1. Major depressive disorders: SSRIs and newer heterocyclics are used in most patients with major depression because they cause fewer side effects and are safer in overdose. TCAs are also effective, but MAOIs are now used infrequently.

   2. Other uses: TCAs and SSRIs are used in bipolar, panic, and phobic disorders.

    a. TCAs are also useful in neuropathic pain and enuresis.

    b. SSRIs are approved for anxiety states, bulimia, obsessive-compulsive disorder, and premenstrual dysphoric disorders (PMDD).

    c. Bupropion is used in withdrawal from nicotine dependence.

E. Toxicities

   1. MAOIs: Overdose results in agitation, hyperthermia, comatose state, and seizures. Hypertensive reactions may occur following ingestion of tyramine-containing foods.

2. **TCAs:** Overdose causes hyperpyrexia, respiratory depression, hypotension, coma, cardiac arrhythmias, and convulsions—the "3 Cs."
3. **SSRIs:** A serotonin syndrome may occur when SSRIs are used with other drugs that increase serotonin effects.
   a. Symptoms include muscle rigidity, hyperthermia, cardiovascular instability, and seizures.
   b. Drugs implicated include MAOIs and TCAs.
4. **Heterocyclics:** Amoxapine causes seizures in overdose; maprotiline causes both seizures and cardiotoxicity.

SUICIDAL IDEATION

The FDA has recently issued warning statements alerting health care providers to an increased risk of suicidality (suicidal thinking and behavior) in children and adolescents being treated with antidepressant drugs.

X. Opioid Analgesics

A. **Concepts**
   1. Receptors for endogenous opioid peptides (eg, enkephalins and endorphins) of multiple subtypes (**mu** [μ], **kappa** [κ], and **delta** [δ]) are targets for opioid analgesic drugs.
   2. Most opioids are nonselective receptor activators, classified as strong, partial, or weak agonists based on analgesic efficacy. **Naloxone** and **naltrexone** block mu (μ) receptors.
   3. Mixed agonist–antagonists (**nalbuphine** and **pentazocine**) activate kappa (κ) receptors but block mu (μ) receptors.

B. **Drug Subclasses and Pharmacokinetics**
   1. **Subclasses: Morphine** (prototype), **meperidine, methadone,** and **fentanyl** are strong agonists; **codeine, oxycodone,** and **hydrocodone** are moderate agonists; **propoxyphene** is a weak agonist (Table 5–8).
   2. **Pharmacokinetics:** Oral bioavailability is limited with morphine due to first-pass metabolism. Opioid analgesics are usually inactivated via metabolism. Morphine forms an active 6-glucuronide metabolite and codeine is partly converted to morphine. Meperidine is metabolized to normeperidine, which causes seizures if accumulated. Duration of analgesic effects range from 1–2 hours (fentanyl) to 6–8 hours (**buprenorphine**).

C. **Mechanisms of Action**
   1. In terms of analgesia, opioids exert both spinal and supraspinal actions.
   2. **Spinal analgesia** occurs by activation of presynaptic opioid receptors, leading to decreased Ca^{2+} influx and decreased release of neurotransmitters involved in nociception (Figure 5–8).
   3. **Supraspinal analgesia** occurs by activation of postsynaptic opioid receptors in the medulla and midbrain, causing inhibition of neurons involved in pain pathways via increased flux of K^+ ions.

D. **Pharmacodynamics**
   1. **Analgesia:** Efficacy is variable depending on the drug.
   2. **Sedation:** Strong agonists cause more sedation (euphoria).
   3. **Respiratory depression:** Increased PCO_2 causes cerebral vasodilation; decreased respiratory drive is the cause of death in overdose.

Table 5–8. Characteristics of selected opioid analgesics.

Drug	Receptors	Analgesia	Respiratory Depression	Abuse Liability	Other Characteristics
Morphine	Strong mu (μ) agonist	+++	Marked	Marked	Releases histamine; poor oral bioavailability
Meperidine	Strong mu (μ) agonist	+++	Marked	Marked	Muscarinic receptor blocker
Methadone	Strong mu (μ) agonist	+++	Marked	Marked	Used in withdrawal states
Oxycodone	Moderate mu (μ) agonist	++	Moderate	Moderate	Potential overdose toxicity with extended-release formulations
Codeine	Moderate mu (μ) agonist	++	Moderate	Moderate	Additive analgesia with aspirin and acetaminophen
Propoxyphene	Weak mu (μ) agonist	+/–	Mild	Moderate	Overdose toxicity and withdrawal signs
Nalbuphine	Kappa (k) agonist, mu (μ) antagonist	++(+)	Moderate	Moderate	Overdose toxicity may not respond to naloxone
Pentazocine	Kappa (k) agonist, mu (μ) antagonist	++	Mild	Minimal	May impede analgesic action of strong mu (μ) agonist

4. **Cardiovascular:** Cerebral vasodilation may increase intracranial pressure; morphine causes vasodilation via histamine release.
5. **Gastrointestinal:** Decreased peristalsis causes constipation.
6. **Other smooth muscle:** Opioids cause relaxation of uterine smooth muscle and contraction of biliary, bladder, and ureteral smooth muscle (except meperidine).
7. **Pupils:** Opioids (except meperidine) cause miosis.

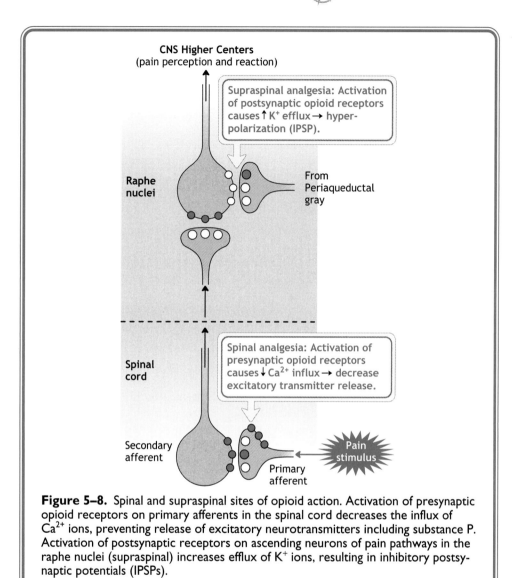

CNS Higher Centers
(pain perception and reaction)

Supraspinal analgesia: Activation of postsynaptic opioid receptors causes ↑K⁺ efflux → hyper-polarization (IPSP).

**Raphe
nuclei**

From
Periaqueductal
gray

Spinal analgesia: Activation of presynaptic opioid receptors causes ↓Ca^{2+} influx → decrease excitatory transmitter release.

**Spinal
cord**

Secondary
afferent

Pain
stimulus

Primary
afferent

Figure 5–8. Spinal and supraspinal sites of opioid action. Activation of presynaptic opioid receptors on primary afferents in the spinal cord decreases the influx of Ca^{2+} ions, preventing release of excitatory neurotransmitters including substance P. Activation of postsynaptic receptors on ascending neurons of pain pathways in the raphe nuclei (supraspinal) increases efflux of K⁺ ions, resulting in inhibitory postsynaptic potentials (IPSPs).

8. **Cough suppression:** Opioids have an antitussive effect.
9. **Emesis:** Opioids stimulate the chemoreceptor trigger zone.
10. **Tolerance:** Chronic use leads to marked tolerance to most actions except constipation and miosis.
11. **Dependence:** Psychological and physical dependence occur to an extent determined by both drug and dosage.
   a. Abuse liability is greatest with strong agonists.
   b. On abrupt discontinuance the **withdrawal (abstinence) syndrome** includes yawning, chills, piloerection, rhinorrhea, lacrimation, agitation, severe gastrointestinal cramping, and muscle jerks.

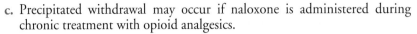

    c. Precipitated withdrawal may occur if naloxone is administered during chronic treatment with opioid analgesics.

  E. **Clinical Uses**

    1. **Analgesia:** Choice of drug is based on analgesic need.

    2. **Cough suppression:** Useful drugs include codeine and dextromethorphan.

    3. **Diarrheal states:** Useful drugs include loperamide and diphenoxylate.

    4. **Anesthesia:** Drugs used include fentanyl and morphine.

    5. **Withdrawal states:** Methadone, with dose tapering, is used to suppress symptoms of opioid withdrawal. Naltrexone is used to decrease craving in alcoholism.

MORPHINE AND PULMONARY EDEMA

CLINICAL CORRELATION

- *In addition to nitroglycerine and loop diuretics, morphine has been used in cardiogenic pulmonary edema because its vasodilating actions may reduce preload.*
- *Although its anxiolytic actions may be beneficial, there is little evidence that morphine provides significant direct hemodynamic effects and the potential adverse effects of the drug, including respiratory depression, may outweigh its usefulness.*
- *Low doses of benzodiazepines are commonly preferred to alleviate anxiety in patients with pulmonary edema.*

  F. **Toxicity**

    1. **Overdose** may result in coma with marked respiratory depression and hypotension, necessitating the use of naloxone.

    2. **Interactions** include additive CNS depression with other drugs including alcohol. Meperidine is implicated in hypertensive crisis with MAO inhibitors, and the serotonin syndrome with SSRIs.

 XI. **Drugs of Abuse**

  A. **Concepts and Drug Categories**

    1. **Drug abuse** is the use of an illicit drug or the excessive or nonmedical use of a licit drug. Occurrence of a withdrawal syndrome on discontinuance acts as reinforcement for continued abuse.

    2. **Abused drugs** include cocaine, amphetamine and derivatives, sedative-hypnotics (including ethanol), heroin and other opioid analgesics, **marijuana,** hallucinogens, **phencyclidine,** and inhalants (solvents, **nitrous oxide,** and **nitrites**).

  B. **Overdose Toxicities**

    1. **CNS stimulants:** Amphetamines and cocaine cause agitation, hypertension, tachycardia, hyperthermia, mydriasis, arrhythmias, and seizures. Methylene dioxymethamphetamine (MDMA, ecstasy) toxicity resembles amphetamine toxicity.

    2. **Sedative-hypnotics** cause slurred speech, drunken behavior, weak and rapid pulse, clammy skin, shallow respirations, mydriasis, and coma.

    3. **Opioid analgesics** cause miosis, drowsiness, nausea, clammy skin, respiratory depression, and coma.

    4. **Hallucinogens** (LSD and mescaline) cause nausea, weakness, paresthesias, and marked perceptual and psychological symptoms.

    5. **Phencyclidine** causes nystagmus, muscle rigidity, hypertension, and seizures.

6. Inhalants: Nitrous oxide has caused fatalities due to inadequate oxygenation; nitrites elicit reflex tachycardia; and inhaled solvents cause CNS depression, respiratory failure, coma, and organ system toxicity.

CNS DRUGS TO AVOID IN PREGNANCY

- *Drugs known or suspected to cause teratogenic effects include carbamazepine (craniofacial anomalies), ethanol (mental retardation and microcephaly), lithium (cardiac malformations), phenytoin (craniofacial anomalies), and valproic acid (spina bifida).*
- *Drugs that may contribute to depression of neonatal functions, when used near term or during delivery, include anesthetics, opioid analgesics, sedative-hypnotics, and tricyclic antidepressants.*

CLINICAL PROBLEMS

A 30-year-old male patient complains of restlessness, feeling "on edge," difficulty concentrating, and disturbances in his sleep patterns. He has a past history of alcohol abuse and attends meetings of Alcoholics Anonymous. The patient is diagnosed as suffering from generalized anxiety disorder and his physician prescribes a drug that is established to be effective in this disorder, but has minimal abuse liability.

1. Which of the following drugs is appropriate for treatment of this patient?
   A. Alprazolam
   B. Bupropion
   C. Haloperidol
   D. Naltrexone
   E. Paroxetine

After using the prescribed drug for a few weeks, the patient complains of "jitteriness," insomnia, and sexual dysfunction including anorgasmia.

2. Which of the following drugs is an alternative (and appropriate) drug for treatment of generalized anxiety disorder in this patient?
   A. Buspirone
   B. Clomipramine
   C. Clozapine
   D. Diazepam
   E. Trazodone

School performance of a 9-year-old child has been declining for several months due to lack of attentiveness and "daydreaming." The child, of average intelligence, has brief spells of staring into space that last 10 or 15 seconds. They occur several times an hour, but the child seems quite unaware of their occurrence. An EEG reveals frontally predominant, generalized 3-Hz spike-and-wave complexes.

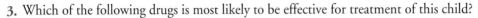

3. Which of the following drugs is most likely to be effective for treatment of this child?

   A. Baclofen

   B. Dantrolene

   C. Ethosuximide

   D. Imipramine

   E. Phenytoin

4. If valproic acid is to be administered to this child, which of the following tests must first be carried out to establish baseline?

   A. Auditory function

   B. Creatinine clearance

   C. Hepatic function

   D. Intelligence quotient

   E. Visual acuity

A 50-year-old female has a long history of treatment with psychiatric drugs for conditions that have required hospitalization on several occasions during the past decade. She presents with stereotypic orolingual and masticatory movements, with involuntary lip-smacking and tongue protrusions.

5. Based on these symptoms she is most likely suffering from which of the following?

   A. Abstinence signs due to abrupt withdrawal from lithium maintenance

   B. Neuroleptic malignant syndrome

   C. Obsessive-compulsive disorder

   D. Tardive dyskinesias

   E. Tourette's syndrome

An irritable and hostile young man is brought to a hospital emergency room by friends who tell the attending physician that he is "withdrawing" from the nonprescription use of a "downer." His signs and symptoms include dehydration, hyperthermia, tachycardia, tachypnea, and hand tremor.

6. If he develops a seizure in the emergency room requiring intravenous lorazepam, he is probably experiencing symptoms of withdrawal from the use of which of the following?

   A. Amitriptyline

   B. Buspirone

   C. Heroin

   D. Methamphetamine

   E. Secobarbital

7. The epidural administration of fentanyl is likely to result in which of the following?

   A. Activation of excitatory glutamate receptors

   B. Demyelination

C. Inhibition of the release of substance P

D. Seizures due to formation of a neurotoxic metabolite

E. Supraspinal analgesia

8. Which of the following statements about the metabolism of neuropharmacologic agents is accurate?

A. Analgesic effects of codeine result from its metabolic conversion to methadone

B. Deficiencies in acetylcholinesterase are responsible for prolonged muscle relaxation with succinylcholine

C. In patients with Parkinson's disease who are using selegiline, a hypertensive crisis occurs following ingestion of cheese and wine

D. Phase II metabolism of morphine leads to the formation of an active metabolite

E. Selective serotonin reuptake inhibitors all form active metabolites with long elimination half-lives

ANSWERS

1. The answer is E.

2. The answer is A. Drugs with no (or minimal) abuse liability that are effective in generalized anxiety disorder (GAD) include buspirone, paroxetine, and venlafaxine. Benzodiazepines such as alprazolam and diazepam, though effective in GAD, would be inappropriate in a patient with a past history of drug abuse. Bupropion and trazodone are heterocyclic antidepressants and clozapine and haloperidol are antipsychotics; none of these drugs has proven efficacy in GAD. Clomipramine, a tricyclic antidepressant, is a back-up drug for obsessive-compulsive disorders. Naltrexone may decrease craving in the management of alcohol dependency, but it is not an anxiolytic drug.

3. The answer is C. The child has several of the characteristic symptoms of absence seizures. A preliminary diagnosis of this condition would be confirmed by the EEG. Ethosuximide and valproic acid have proven efficacy in absence seizures.

4. The answer is C. Anorexia, vomiting, malaise, and lethargy may precede changes in liver function that are characteristic of valproic acid toxicity. Liver function tests should be obtained before treatment with valproic acid and at frequent intervals during the first 6 months of therapy.

5. The answer is D. Tardive dyskinesias are adverse effects that occur during treatment of psychotic states with drugs that block dopamine receptors in the striatum (eg, haloperidol and phenothiazines). These choreoathetoid irregular muscle movements appear to result from sensitization of dopamine receptors. They are not readily reversed on drug discontinuance and are exacerbated by muscarinic blocking agents. A major advantage of newer antipsychotic drugs is that they are much less likely to cause extrapyramidal dysfunction.

6. The answer is E. The young man described is experiencing the symptoms of the withdrawal or abstinence syndrome that follows the development of physical dependence on a sedative-hypnotic drug. The severity of his symptoms is commensurate with the abuse of high doses of a short-acting barbiturate (eg, secobarbital or "reds"). They are similar to those that would occur following abrupt discontinuance of excessive use of alcohol. The symptoms described are quite different from those characteristic of withdrawal following dependence on opioid analgesics (eg, heroin) or CNS stimulants (eg, methamphetamine).

7. The answer is C. Activation of presynaptic opioid receptors on primary afferents by opioid analgesic drugs provides **spinal analgesia** by inhibiting the release of neurotransmitters (including substance P) that are involved in pain responses.

8. The answer is D. Morphine-6-glucuronide has analgesic activity equivalent to that of morphine. Codeine is metabolized to form morphine, not methadone. Prolongation of the action of succinylcholine occurs in patients deficient in nonspecific esterases, not acetylcholinesterase. Hypertensive reactions to tyramine occur in patients using inhibitors of MAO type A; selegiline inhibits the B form of the enzyme. Fluoxetine is the only SSRI that forms a long-acting active metabolite (norfluoxetine).

CHAPTER 6
HORMONES AND OTHER ENDOCRINE AGENTS

I. Hypothalamic and Pituitary Drugs

A. The major hormones produced by the hypothalamus and pituitary gland (Table 6–1) act primarily on cell surface receptors, especially G protein coupled receptors.

B. Clinically useful hypothalamic and pituitary agents are administered parenterally.

   1. **Growth hormone (GH) (somatotropin)**, a protein produced by recombinant DNA technology, is used to treat GH deficiency and Turner's syndrome and to improve growth in children with chronic renal insufficiency. GH has been abused or misused by individuals attempting to bulk up muscles or slow the aging process. **Somatostatin** inhibits GH release.

   2. **Octreotide** is a synthetic octapeptide somatostatin analog that is useful in slowing the progression or reducing the activity of a number of endocrine disorders, including acromegaly, carcinoid, gastrinoma, and glucagonoma.

   3. **Thyroid-stimulating hormone (TSH)** is a peptide occasionally used for diagnostic purposes in thyroid disorders.

   4. **Adrenocorticotropic hormone (ACTH, adrenocorticotropin)**, another peptide, was once widely used to treat allergic and inflammatory conditions, but has been almost completely replaced by **adrenal steroids.** It is still available.

   5. **Gonadotropin-releasing hormone (GnRH)** and several peptide analogs (eg, **leuprolide, goserelin,** and **nafarelin**) are used to treat infertility in women and to treat tumors responsive to reduction of gonadal steroids. These agents stimulate gonadotropin release when given in pulsatile fashion, but powerfully inhibit the pituitary when given continuously or as depot injections.

   6. **Follicle-stimulating hormone (FSH)** and similar peptides (eg, **urofollitropin** and **recombinant follitropins**) are used to treat infertility in both sexes.

   7. **Human recombinant luteinizing hormone (LH, lutropin alfa)**, **human chorionic gonadotropin (hCG)**, a natural product used as a substitute for **LH, recombinant chorionic gonadotropin (choriogonadotropin alfa)**, and **menotropins,** another natural product that combines both FSH and LH activity, are used to treat infertility.

   8. **Oxytocin** by injection stimulates labor or increases uterine contraction after delivery; as a nasal spray oxytocin stimulates milk let-down in lactating women.

   9. **Vasopressin (antidiuretic hormone, ADH)** is used to treat pituitary diabetes insipidus.

Table 6–1. Some hypothalamic, pituitary, and target organ hormones.

Hypothalamic Hormone	Pituitary Hormone	Target Tissue	Target Tissue Hormone
Growth hormone-releasing hormone	Growth hormone	Liver	Somatomedins
Somatostatin	Growth hormone	Liver	Somatomedins
Thyrotropin-releasing hormone	Thyrotropin	Thyroid	Thyroxine
Corticotropin-releasing hormone	Adrenocorticotropic hormone	Adrenal cortex	Glucocorticoids, mineralocorticoids, androgens
Oxytocin	None	Smooth muscle of uterus, ducts of breast	None
Vasopressin	None	Renal tubules, smooth muscle of vessels	None

      a. **Desmopressin,** an ADH analog, is longer acting and more frequently used.
      b. These drugs are not useful in treating **nephrogenic** diabetes insipidus, in which thiazide diuretics are used to reduce urine volume (see Chapter 3).

II. Thyroid Drugs

  A. **Thyroid deficiency** (**hypothyroidism** or **myxedema**) is treated by simple replacement of thyroxine.
    1. **Levothyroxine** (T_4, **thyroxine**) is readily available, well standardized, and inexpensive.
    2. **Triiodothyronine** (T_3, **liothyronine**), with a faster and shorter action, is occasionally used.
    3. These hormones, which are orally active, act chiefly on intracellular receptors that influence gene expression.
  B. **Thyroid overactivity** (**hyperthyroidism**) is treated in several ways. The biosynthesis of thyroid hormones and targets of therapy are shown in Figure 6–1.
    1. **Thioamides** are the most important antithyroid drugs.
      a. **Propylthiouracil** and **methimazole,** both orally active, interfere with incorporation of iodine into thyroglobulin and possibly block coupling of the monomers monoiodotyrosine and diiodotyrosine to form thyroxine and triiodothyronine.
      b. **Toxicity** includes rash, hypoprothrombinemia, and agranulocytosis.
    2. **Radioactive iodine** (^{131}I) is an effective treatment for thyrotoxicosis.
      a. Because it is avidly taken up by the thyroid (thereby sparing other tissues), the radiation emitted by the isotope is sufficient to destroy most or all of the gland.
      b. Most patients are then maintained on **levothyroxine.**

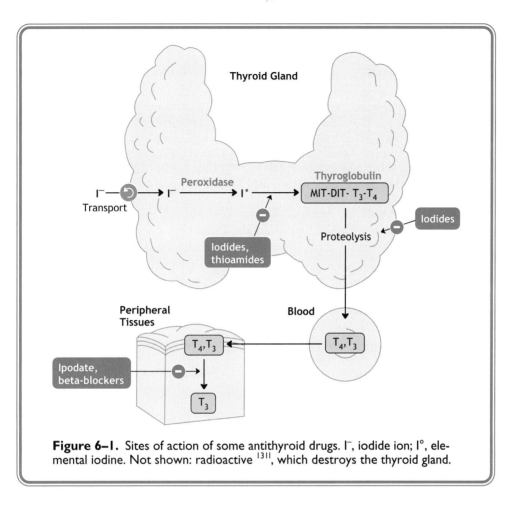

Figure 6–1. Sites of action of some antithyroid drugs. I⁻, iodide ion; I°, elemental iodine. Not shown: radioactive ¹³¹I, which destroys the thyroid gland.

3. **Iodinated radiocontrast media** (eg, **ipodate**), provides rapid and effective treatment of thyroid storm by reducing the release of thyroxine from the gland and blocking the conversion of thyroxine to triiodothyronine.
4. **Iodide salts and iodine** inhibit the incorporation of iodine into the thyroglobulin molecule, inhibit the release of thyroxine from the gland, and are especially useful in reducing vascularity of the gland before thyroidectomy.
5. **β Blockers** (eg, **propranolol**) are very useful in the management of thyroid storm. Propranolol controls tachycardia and other arrhythmias associated with hyperthyroidism and inhibits the conversion of thyroxine into triiodothyronine.

III. Adrenal Steroids and Antagonists

A. Mechanisms of Action

1. **Steroid receptors:** Corticosteroids bind to cytosolic receptors and the complexes formed undergo dimerization and then enter the cell nucleus. There they alter gene expression by binding to tissue-specific nuclear response elements.

2. **Metabolic effects:** Glucocorticoids increase gluconeogenesis, insulin secretion, and both lipogenesis and lipolysis.

   a. Catabolic effects include wasting of muscle protein and lymphoid tissue, osteoporosis, and growth inhibition.

   b. Mineralocorticoids increase synthesis of ion transporters and Na^+ channels in the renal collecting tubules.

3. **Immunosuppressive and anti-inflammatory actions:** Glucocorticoids inhibit some of the mechanisms involved in cell-mediated immunologic functions.

   a. High doses of glucocorticoids result in decreased synthesis of prostaglandins and leukotrienes via inhibition of phospholipase A_2, decreased mRNA of COX-2, decreased platelet-activating factor (PAF), and decreased synthesis of interleukin 2 (IL-2).

   b. Cellular consequences include decreased leukocyte migration, decreased phagocytosis, stabilization of capillary permeability, and decreased lymphocyte proliferation and activation.

B. **Drugs & Pharmacokinetics**

1. **Natural corticosteroids: Cortisol,** the major natural glucocorticoid, is rapidly metabolized and has a short duration of action if used orally.

   a. Cortisol has significant mineralocorticoid effects.

   b. **Aldosterone** is the major natural mineralocorticoid.

2. **Synthetic corticosteroids:** Synthetic glucocorticoids have longer durations of action and less mineralocorticoid effect than cortisol.

   a. **Prednisone, triamcinolone,** and **dexamethasone** (in order of increasing duration of action) are synthetic glucocorticoids.

   b. **Fludrocortisone** is a synthetic mineralocorticoid.

C. **Clinical Uses**

1. **Adrenal dysfunction:** Glucocorticoids and mineralocorticoids are used as replacement therapy in Addison's disease and as supplementation in acute adrenal insufficiency states (infection, shock, and trauma).

2. **Nonendocrine uses:** Glucocorticoids are used to treat a wide range of inflammatory and immune disorders including asthma, cancer, collagen diseases, organ transplant rejection, rheumatoid arthritis, and systemic lupus erythematosus, and to prevent the neonatal respiratory distress syndrome associated with premature delivery.

PHARMACOLOGIC VERSUS PHYSIOLOGIC DRUG ACTIONS

CLINICAL CORRELATION

- *Endocrine pharmacology illustrates the marked differences between low (physiologic) and high (pharmacologic) doses of drugs.*
- *Replacement therapy in hormone deficiency states involves use of physiologic doses of hormones and consequently adverse effects are not usually severe.*
- *In inflammatory or immunologic disorders pharmacologic doses of steroids are usually needed and adverse effects are sometimes severe.*

D. **Toxicities**

1. The **suppression of ACTH** results in adrenocortical atrophy.

2. A **cushingoid state** involves fat deposition and muscle atrophy.

3. **Metabolic effects** of glucocorticoids include hyperglycemia and increased insulin demand (diabetogenic action), osteoporosis, aseptic hip necrosis, and de-

creased skeletal growth in children. Drugs with mineralocorticoid activity may cause electrolyte imbalance, edema, and hypertension.

2. Other toxicities include gastrointestinal ulcers, decreased wound healing, cataract formation, glaucoma, increased infections, and mental dysfunction.

E. **Corticosteroid Antagonists**

1. Receptor antagonists: Spironolactone blocks aldosterone receptors (see Chapter 3, section on diuretics). **Mifepristone,** a progestin receptor antagonist, also blocks glucocorticoid receptors and has been used in Cushing's syndrome.

2. Synthesis inhibitors: Ketoconazole, which inhibits synthesis of both corticosteroids and gonadal steroids, is used in adrenal carcinoma, breast cancer, and hirsutism. **Metyrapone,** which inhibits 11-hydroxylation, is used diagnostically in tests of adrenal function.

IV. Gonadal Drugs, Antagonists, and Inhibitors

A. **Mechanisms**

1. Natural gonadal hormones include the **estrogens, progestins,** and **androgens.**

a. Multiple endocrine functions result from binding of the hormones to specific intracellular receptors in responsive tissues.

b. Interaction of such hormone–receptor complexes with nuclear response elements leads to modulation of gene transcription, resulting in tissue-specific actions.

2. Agents that modify the natural functions of gonadal hormones do so by activation or antagonism of their receptors or by inhibition of hormone synthesis. The sites of action of ovarian hormones and their analogs are shown in Figure 6–2.

B. **Drug Classes**

1. Estrogens include **estradiol** (natural), **conjugated equine estrogens, ethinyl estradiol, mestranol,** and **diethylstilbestrol** (nonsteroidal).

2. Agents influencing estrogen activity include **tamoxifen** and **raloxifene** (selective estrogen receptor modulators, SERMs), **clomiphene** (a partial agonist), and **anastrozole** (an aromatase inhibitor).

3. Progestins include **medroxyprogesterone, norethindrone,** and **norgestrel,** which are receptor activators; **mifepristone** is a receptor antagonist.

4. Androgens include **methyltestosterone** and anabolic steroids (eg, **oxandrolone**).

5. Antiandrogens include **flutamide** (a receptor antagonist), **finasteride** (a 5α-reductase inhibitor), **ketoconazole** (a synthesis inhibitor), and **leuprolide** (a GnRH analog).

SELECTIVE ESTROGEN RECEPTOR MODULATORS (SERMS)

- *SERMs activate estrogen (E) receptors in some tissues, but act as partial agonists or antagonists in others.*
- *Tamoxifen antagonizes E receptors in breast tissue, but activates E receptors in endometrial tissue.*
- *Raloxifene activates E receptors in bone, but antagonizes E receptors in breast and endometrial tissues.*

C. **Clinical Applications**

1. Clinical uses of estrogens, progestins, and antagonists are given in Table 6–2.

2. Clinical uses of androgens and antagonists are given in Table 6–3.

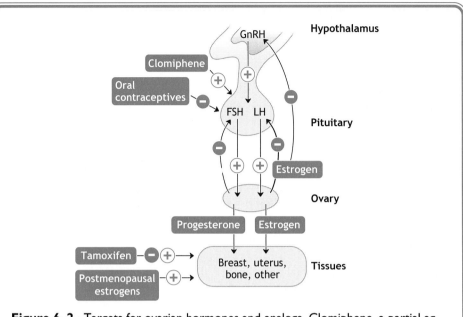

Figure 6–2. Targets for ovarian hormones and analogs. Clomiphene, a partial agonist, is mainly an antagonist at pituitary estrogen receptors; this prevents negative feedback and increases the output of the pituitary gonadotropic hormones. Tamoxifen, a SERM (see text), is mainly an antagonist at estrogen receptors in the breast, but acts as an agonist in bone. Contraceptives reduce FSH and LH output from the pituitary by activating feedback receptors.

D. Toxicities

1. **Estrogens** cause nausea, breast tenderness, endometrial hyperplasia, migraine, thromboembolic phenomena, gallbladder disease, and hypertriglyceridemia; in pregnancy diethylstilbestrol has caused vaginal adenocarcinoma in offspring.
2. **Progestins** result in acne, decreased high-density lipoprotein (HDL)-cholesterol, depression, hirsutism, and weight gain.
3. **Androgens** result in masculinization (feminization in high doses), premature closure of the epiphyses, cholestatic jaundice, and mental changes.

FEEDBACK INHIBITION IN ENDOCRINE PHARMACOLOGY

Feedback inhibition *is the principle underlying the contraceptive actions of ovarian hormones. Ovarian hormones interact with receptors on cells in the hypothalamus and/or anterior pituitary to prevent ovulation by inhibiting the release of GnRH and the pituitary gonadotropins FSH and LH.*

V. Pancreatic Drugs

A. Concepts

1. **Insulin** is a polypeptide produced from proinsulin and released from **pancreatic beta cells** by **insulinogens** including glucose.

Table 6–2. Clinical uses of estrogens, progestins, and antagonists.

Clinical Use	Drugs
Female hypogonadism	Conjugated estrogens, ethinyl estradiol
Hormone replacement therapy; osteoporosis	Estrogens and progestins (the combination decreases endometrial hyperplasia); raloxifene
Contraception (feedback inhibition of pituitary FSH and LH)	*Oral*[1]: combinations of estrogens and progestins, or progestins alone *Parenteral:* medroxyprogesterone (IM), or combinations of estrogens and progestins as transdermal patch or vaginal ring
Dysmenorrhea and uterine bleeding	Estrogens, GnRH analogs, progestins
Infertility	Clomiphene, a partial agonist at pituitary E receptors, increases FSH and LH); GnRH analogs
Abortifacients	Mifepristone (progestin antagonist) and prostaglandin
Endometriosis	Oral contraceptives, GnRH analogs, danazole (inhibits ovarian hormone synthesis)
Breast cancer	Tamoxifen (estrogen receptor antagonism); anastrozole (aromatase inhibitor)

[1]Oral contraceptives decrease the incidence of endometrial and ovarian cancer, dysmenorrhea, endometriosis, and pelvic inflammatory disease.

    a. The major targets for insulin are liver (increased glucose uptake and storage as glycogen), muscle (increased glucose uptake and increased synthesis of glycogen and protein), and adipose tissue (increased glucose uptake and triglyceride storage and decreased lipolysis).

    b. Insulin receptors in these tissues function as transmembrane tyrosine kinases.

  2. Diabetes mellitus results from a deficiency of insulin and/or decreased sensitivity of target tissues to its actions.

    a. Management strategies include use of insulin and oral antidiabetic drugs and the control of diet, weight, and blood pressure.

    b. Patients with type 1 diabetes have an absolute requirement for insulin.

 B. Insulin Forms & Toxicities

  1. Insulin forms: Human insulin for subcutaneous administration is available in multiple forms that differ in their onset, time to peak effects, and duration of action.

Table 6–3. Clinical uses of androgens and antagonists.

Clinical Use	Drugs
Male hypogonadism	Testosterone derivatives (oral, patch), methyltestosterone
Anabolic protein synthesis	Nandrolone, oxandrolone
Benign prostatic hyperplasia	Finasteride (also used in male pattern baldness)
Prostate carcinoma	Flutamide, leuprolide, ketoconazole
Hirsutism	Flutamide, oral contraceptives, spironolactone

     a. Rapid-onset, short-acting forms used to control postprandial hyperglycemia include **insulin lispro** (peak < 0.5 hour) and **regular zinc insulin.**

     b. Maintenance forms (**NPH** and **lente insulins**) vary in time to peak activity (4–12 hours) and duration (18–24 hours).

     c. **Insulin glargine,** the longest-acting form (> 24 hours), has no peak.

  2. **Insulin toxicities: Hypoglycemia** from insulin overdose may require prompt use of oral or parenteral glucose or glucagon by intramuscular injection.

     a. Children, the elderly, and patients with nephropathy are most susceptible to hypoglycemia.

     b. Local reactions at injection sites include redness, swelling, and itching.

     c. Systemic allergies (rare) may result in severe rashes and possible anaphylaxis.

DIABETIC KETOACIDOSIS (DKA)

*Prolonged **hyperglycemia**, resulting most commonly from missed or inadequate doses of insulin, causes anorexia, thirst, flushing, tachycardia, acetone smell of the breath, Kussmaul's respirations, and acidosis. The condition may be life-threatening and necessitates intravenous treatment with rapid-onset forms of insulin and meticulous management of electrolyte and acid–base derangements.*

  C. Sulfonylureas

    1. **Mechanisms: Sulfonylureas** are oral hypoglycemic agents that block K^+ channels in pancreatic beta cell membranes, resulting in the opening of voltage-regulated Ca^{2+} channels.

     a. The influx of Ca^{2+} elicits release of insulin from storage vesicles (Figure 6–3).

     b. Glucagon release from pancreatic alpha cells is inhibited and subsequently both muscle and liver cells increase their sensitivity to insulin.

    2. **Drugs and pharmacokinetics:** There are two groups of sulfonylureas.

     a. Older sulfonylureas (eg, **chlorpropamide** and **tolbutamide**) have variable durations of action (6–60 hours), are both metabolized and eliminated unchanged in the urine, and can be displaced from plasma proteins by many drugs with enhancement of hypoglycemic actions.

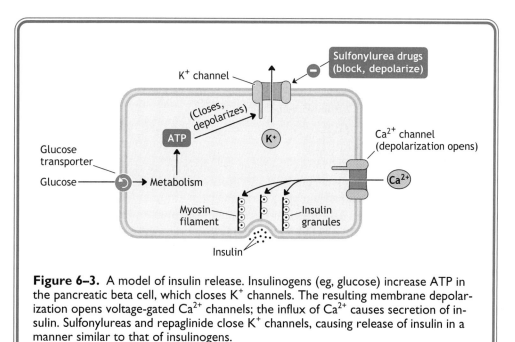

Figure 6–3. A model of insulin release. Insulinogens (eg, glucose) increase ATP in the pancreatic beta cell, which closes K^+ channels. The resulting membrane depolarization opens voltage-gated Ca^{2+} channels; the influx of Ca^{2+} causes secretion of insulin. Sulfonylureas and repaglinide close K^+ channels, causing release of insulin in a manner similar to that of insulinogens.

  b. Newer sulfonylureas (eg, **glimepiride, glipizide,** and **glyburide**) have durations of action from 10–24 hours and are not displaced from plasma proteins.
  3. Clinical uses: Sulfonylureas are used in type 2 diabetes as monotherapy and in combinations with other drugs, including insulin.
  4. Toxicities: Hypoglycemia and weight gain are common and rashes and other allergic reactions are rare.
 D. Thiazolidinediones
  1. Mechanisms: Thiazolidinediones stimulate peroxisome proliferator-activated receptors (PPARs) involved in transcription of insulin-responsive genes, resulting in sensitization of target tissues to insulin, with increased **glucose uptake** and decreased **gluconeogenesis.**
  2. Drugs and clinical uses: Pioglitazone and **rosiglitazone** reduce both fasting and postprandial hyperglycemia and are used quite commonly in type 2 diabetes as monotherapy, or in combinations with other drugs including insulin.
  3. Toxicities: Hypoglycemia is rare, but weight gain is common. Pioglitazone may increase drug metabolism via induction of cytochrome P-450 and can reduce serum concentrations of oral contraceptives and cyclosporine.
 E. Other Oral Antidiabetic Drugs
  1. Metformin reduces postprandial and fasting glucose levels by unknown mechanisms.
   a. The drug is not an insulin secretagogue and does not cause hypoglycemia.
   b. Gastrointestinal distress occurs and there is potential for lactic acidosis.

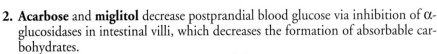

2. **Acarbose** and **miglitol** decrease postprandial blood glucose via inhibition of α-glucosidases in intestinal villi, which decreases the formation of absorbable carbohydrates.
    a. Adverse effects include gastrointestinal distress.
    b. Hypoglycemia does not occur.
3. **Repaglinide** is a short-acting meglitinide that releases insulin by the same mechanism as sulfonylureas.

F. Glucagon
    1. **Source and effects: Glucagon** is a peptide produced by pancreatic alpha cells. Activation of glucagon receptors (G protein coupled) results in an increase in cyclic AMP and leads to hepatic **glycogenolysis** and **gluconeogenesis,** cardiac stimulation, and relaxation of smooth muscle.
    2. **Clinical uses:** Glucagon is used in the treatment of hypoglycemia, reversal of β blocker overdose, and relaxation of the bowel for x-ray visualization.

VI. **Drugs That Affect Bone Mineral Metabolism**

A. **Calcium** and **phosphate** are the most important components of bone mineral. Their levels in the blood are controlled tightly by parathyroid hormone and vitamin D, and less tightly by calcitonin, glucocorticoids, and estrogen.

B. **Parathyroid hormone** (**PTH**) is a large peptide synthesized in the parathyroid glands contained in the thyroid.
    1. It acts via a G protein coupled receptor to increase calcium reabsorption from the urine and from bone.
    2. It increases blood calcium.

C. **Vitamin D** is a secosteroid formed in the skin from vitamin D precursor molecules.
    1. It is commonly used as a food supplement, especially in milk.
    2. Active metabolites formed in the liver and kidney increase intestinal calcium and phosphate absorption and decrease renal excretion. They increase the blood levels of both ions.

D. **Calcitonin,** a peptide secreted by the thyroid, decreases bone resorption and thus decreases blood calcium and phosphate. Injectable and nasal spray preparations of salmon calcitonin are available for acute reduction of serum calcium. Chronic use impairs bone formation.

E. **Estrogens** are important in maintaining bone density in premenopausal women.
    1. Estrogen loss makes postmenopausal women more susceptible to osteoporosis.
    2. Prevention of osteoporosis is an indication for estrogen replacement therapy in postmenopausal women.

F. **Bisphosphonates** (**alendronate, etidronate, pamidronate,** and **risedronate**) are organic polyphosphate molecules that stabilize bone crystal structure and reduce bone resorption.
    1. The older bisphosphonates (eg, **etidronate** and **pamidronate**) reduce bone formation but are effective in the prevention of postmenopausal osteoporosis and fractures.
    2. Newer bisphosphonates (eg, **alendronate**) increase bone formation, and are commonly used for treatment of osteoporosis (postmenopausal and glucocorticoid induced) and for Paget's disease. Alendronate may cause esophageal ulceration if not taken with ample water.

G. **Fluoride ion (F⁻)** is uniquely effective in strengthening the hydroxyapatite crystal of tooth enamel and is indicated as a water additive for the prevention of dental caries in children.
  1. It is not clear whether fluoride increases bone strength in patients at risk for osteoporosis.
  2. In toxic dosages fluoride increases bone formation in ectopic sites (eg, soft tissues).

CLINICAL PROBLEMS

A patient with severe hyperthyroidism presents to the emergency department with cardiac arrhythmia, hyperthermia, delirium, and shock.

1. Which of the following drugs would **not** be considered for his treatment?
   A. Iodide ion in solution
   B. Propranolol
   C. Propylthiouracil
   D. Norepinephrine
   E. Ipodate radiocontrast medium

A man presents for evaluation of infertility. Examination reveals low testosterone level, small testes, and a very low sperm count.

2. Appropriate therapy might include which of the following?
   A. Desmopressin
   B. Leuprolide, given as a long-lasting depot injection
   C. Menotropins
   D. Octreotide
   E. Thyroxine

An 80-year-old man has had three fractures during the past 2 years. A bone density scan reveals significant thinning of his bone.

3. The most appropriate therapy for this patient would be which of the following?
   A. Alendronate
   B. Estrogen
   C. Fluoride
   D. Parathyroid hormone
   E. Vitamin D

A patient with systemic lupus erythematosus (SLE) who has been treated with anti-inflammatory drugs abruptly develops nausea and vomiting, abdominal pain, hyperthermia, and unexplained shock refractory to fluids and pressors. Serum levels of sodium and cortisol are below normal values.

4. Which explanation of these signs and symptoms is most likely?

   A. Abrupt withdrawal from the use of glucocorticoids

   B. Development of heart failure due to excessive use of nonsteroidal anti-inflammatory drugs

   C. Exacerbation of SLE symptoms

   D. Excessive mineralocorticoid effects of steroids

   E. The patient has developed Cushing's syndrome

Drug therapy is being considered for treatment of benign prostatic hyperplasia (BPH) in a 63-year-old man.

5. Which of the following statements about the proposed management of this patient is accurate?

   A. Baseline prostate-specific antigen (PSA) must be determined before drug treatment

   B. Treatment with doxazosin will prevent formation of dihydrotestosterone

   C. Estrogens are drugs of choice in BPH

   D. Finasteride relieves the symptoms of BPH via its activation of α adrenoceptors

   E. In repository form, leuprolide decreases circulating gonadotropins

A patient with type 2 diabetes maintained on an oral agent develops symptoms that include sweating, dizziness, palpitations, tremors, and tingling in the hands and the lips.

6. If these symptoms are drug-related, the most likely causative agent is which of the following?

   A. Acarbose

   B. Glyburide

   C. Prednisone

   D. Metformin

   E. Thiazides

A prescription for oral contraceptives is being considered for a 35-year-old patient.

7. Which of the following medical conditions is least likely to be a relative contraindication?

   A. Depression

   B. Gallbladder disease

   C. Hypertension

   D. Migraine

   E. Pelvic inflammatory disease

Several different drugs are used to reduce the pain and other symptoms associated with endometriosis.

8. Which of the following statements is inaccurate?

    A. Danazole inhibits the midcycle surge of FSH and LH

    B. Leuprolide causes downregulation of pituitary gonadotropin secretion

    C. Symptoms of endometriosis are exacerbated by use of oral contraceptives

    D. Medroxyprogesterone causes endometrial decidualization and atrophy

    E. Pharmacologic agents do not cure endometriosis

ANSWERS

1. The answer is D. All of the drugs listed are appropriate except norepinephrine. Sympathetic activity is abnormally high in thyroid storm and norepinephrine would exacerbate arrhythmias and shock.

2. The answer is C. Menotropins are often used in treating infertility because they combine FSH and LH activity. The other drugs listed are of no value in infertility.

3. The answer is A. A bisphosphonate such as alendronate would be the most appropriate therapy because it increases bone mineral density. Estrogen is inappropriate because the patient is a man. Fluoride, parathyroid hormone, and vitamin D have not been shown to decrease fractures.

4. The answer is A. The patient is suffering from adrenal crisis. Secondary adrenocortical insufficiency occurs when exogenous steroids that have suppressed the pituitary–adrenal axis are withdrawn too rapidly. Dose tapering is mandatory.

5. The answer is E. Baseline prostate-specific antigen (PSA) is nearly always elevated in benign prostatic hyperplasia (BPH) and is not a requirement for drug treatment. Doxazosin is an α blocker; finasteride inhibits 5α-reductase, decreasing dihydrotestosterone. Estrogens are rarely acceptable for use in BPH. Leuprolide (a GnRH analog), when used in repository form decreases gonadotropins, resulting in decreased synthesis of androgens.

6. The answer is B. The symptoms experienced by this patient with diabetes are typical of hypoglycemia. Glucocorticoids and thiazide diuretics cause hyperglycemia, resulting in an increased need for insulin. Acarbose which decreases postprandial glucose and metformin rarely cause hypoglycemic reactions. Newer sulfonylureas (eg, glyburide) are potent releasers of insulin and often cause hypoglycemia.

7. The answer is E. The estrogen components of oral contraceptives are associated with exacerbation of gallbladder disease and migraine attacks. Progestin components may cause severe depression, often a reason for discontinuance of oral contraceptive use. In a 35-year-old hypertensive patient oral contraceptives increase the risk of thromboembolic phenomena.

8. The answer is C. Drug management can alleviate the symptoms of endometriosis, but is not curative. Oral contraceptives, progestins, gonadotropin-releasing hormone analogs, and danazole are all effective in the symptomatic management of this common disorder.

CHAPTER 7
ANTIMICROBIAL AGENTS: ANTIBIOTICS

I. Inhibitors of Cell Wall Synthesis: Penicillins

A. Classification

1. **Penicillins** are bactericidal antibiotics that contain a β-lactam ring structure that must be intact for antibacterial activity.

2. **Subclasses** of penicillins differ in antimicrobial activities and susceptibility to inactivation by microbial enzymes that break the ring structure (β-lactamases).

    a. **Penicillinase-susceptible narrow-spectrum** drugs include **penicillin G** and **penicillin V**.

    b. **Penicillinase-resistant narrow-spectrum** drugs include **methicillin** and **nafcillin**.

    c. **Penicillinase-susceptible wider-spectrum** drugs include **ampicillin, amoxicillin,** and **ticarcillin.**

B. Mechanisms

1. **Mechanisms of action:** Penicillins bind to specific proteins (penicillin-binding proteins, PBPs) on bacterial cytoplasmic membranes and inhibit transpeptidation, the final step in cell wall synthesis (Figure 7–1), and also activate autolytic enzymes, which cause lesions in the bacterial cell membrane and wall.

2. **Mechanisms of resistance:** There are three primary mechanisms that result in loss of antibacterial activity.

    a. Formation of penicillinases (eg, by staphylococci and gram-negative bacilli) is a major mechanism of bacterial resistance.

    b. Changes in PBP structure prevent binding (eg, that seen in methicillin-resistant *Staphylococcus aureus* [MRSA], also called nafcillin-resistant *Staphylococcus aureus* [NRSA], and penicillin-resistant *Streptococcus pneumoniae* [PRSP]).

    c. Changes in porin structure prevent access to the cytoplasmic membrane (eg, that seen in *Pseudomonas* strains resistant to ticarcillin).

C. Pharmacokinetics

1. **Oral bioavailability:** Gastric acid inactivates some penicillins (eg, penicillin G).

2. **Elimination:** Most penicillins are eliminated via active tubular secretion with half-lives of less than 60 minutes; nafcillin is eliminated in the bile and ampicillin undergoes enterohepatic cycling.

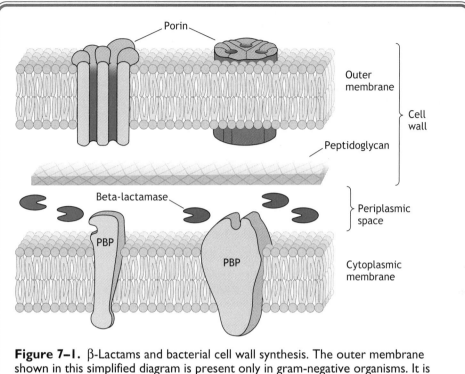

Figure 7–1. β-Lactams and bacterial cell wall synthesis. The outer membrane shown in this simplified diagram is present only in gram-negative organisms. It is penetrated by proteins (porins) that are permeable to hydrophilic substances such as β-lactam antibiotics. The peptidoglycan chains (mureins) are cross-linked by transpeptidases located in the cytoplasmic membrane, closely associated with penicillin-binding proteins (PBPs). β-Lactam antibiotics bind to PBPs and inhibit transpeptidation, the final step in cell wall synthesis. They also activate autolytic enzymes that cause lesions in the cell wall. β-Lactamases, which inactivate β-lactam antibiotics, may be present in the periplasmic space or on the outer surface of the cytoplasmic membrane. (Reproduced, with permission, from Katzung BG [editor]: *Basic & Clinical Pharmacology,* 9th ed. McGraw-Hill, 2004.)

      3. Repository form: Benzathine penicillin G has a half-life of more than 14 days.

  D. Clinical Uses

      1. The clinical uses of penicillins depend on the subclass to which the penicillin belongs.

      2. Table 7–1 lists the clinical uses of various penicillins.

  E. Toxicities

      1. There is a wide range of **hypersensitivity** reactions with a 5–6% incidence. Assume complete cross-allergenicity between different penicillins.

      2. Gastrointestinal reactions include nausea and diarrhea as well as potential opportunistic infections by fungi (upper gastrointestinal [GI]) or bacteria (antibiotic-associated colitis).

      3. Maculopapular rash is a reaction to ampicillin.

Table 7–1. Clinical uses of penicillins.

Penicillin	Infections
Penicillin G	Common streptococci, pneumococci (if susceptible), enterococci (synergy with aminoglycosides), meningococci, *Treponema pallidum* (drug of choice), and related spirochetes
Nafcillin, oxacillin, and related drugs	Known or suspected staphylococcal infections (not MRSA)
Amoxicillin and ampicillin	Susceptible streptococci, *Escherichia coli*, *Haemophilus influenzae*, *Moraxella catarrhalis*, *Listeria monocytogenes*, and *Helicobacter pylori*
Ticarcillin and related drugs	Gram-negative bacilli including *Pseudomonas aeruginosa* (synergy with aminoglycosides)

PENICILLINASE INHIBITORS

- *The antibacterial activities of certain penicillins are enhanced by their administration together with chemicals such as clavulanic acid and sulbactam.*
- *These compounds act as suicide inhibitors of bacterial penicillinases.*
- *Amoxicillin, a penicillinase-susceptible drug, has activity against strains of staphylococci that produce penicillinases when used in combination with clavulanic acid.*
- *Likewise, the activity of ticarcillin against certain gram-negative bacilli is enhanced if it is administered together with sulbactam, a penicillinase inhibitor.*

II. Inhibitors of Cell Wall Synthesis: Cephalosporins, Carbapenems, and Vancomycin

A. Cephalosporins

1. **Mechanisms:** Cephalosporins are bactericidal β-lactams with mechanisms of action identical to the penicillins. Resistance may occur via β-lactamase (cephalosporinase) formation and changes in PBPs.
2. **Classification:** There are four generations of cephalosporins that differ in their antibacterial spectrum and pharmacokinetics (Table 7–2).
3. **Pharmacokinetics:** Most cephalosporins are eliminated via active tubular secretion with half-lives of 1–2 hours.
   a. **Cefoperazone** and **ceftriaxone** are eliminated in the bile.
   b. First- and second-generation drugs do not enter the central nervous system (CNS).
   c. Third-generation drugs can provide cerebrospinal fluid (CSF) levels adequate for treatment of bacterial meningitis.

Table 7–2. Clinical uses of cephalosporins.

Cephalosporins	Infections
First-generation: **cefazolin, cephalexin**	Gram-positive cocci (not MRSA), *Escherichia coli*, *Klebsiella pneumoniae*, and some *Proteus* species
Second-generation: **cefotetan, cefaclor**	Gram-negative bacilli including *Bacteroides fragilis* (cefotetan); *Haemophilus influenzae* and *Moraxella catarrhalis* (cefaclor)
Third-generation	Many gram-positive and gram-negative cocci and gram-negative bacilli including ß-lactamase–forming strains; individual drugs have activity against specific organisms including *Pseudomonas* (**ceftazidime**), anaerobes (**ceftizoxime**), and gonococci (**ceftriaxone, cefixime**)
Fourth-generation	**Cefipime** combines the gram-positive activity of the first-generation drugs with the gram-negative activity of the third-generation drugs

    B. Clinical Uses
       1. Clinical uses of cephalosporins vary depending on the generation of the drug.
       2. Table 7–2 lists the clinical uses of cephalosporins.

LIMITATIONS OF CEPHALOSPORINS

- *The third- and fourth-generation cephalosporins have a wide spectrum of antibacterial action that includes many significant pathogens.*
- *However, there are gaps in the antibacterial activity of cephalosporins that are noteworthy.*
- *None of the cephalosporins has clinically useful activity in the treatment of infections caused by methicillin-resistant staphylococci, Listeria species, enterococci, Mycoplasma pneumoniae, or chlamydia.*

    C. Toxicities
       1. There is a wide range of allergic reactions, with a 1–2% incidence.
         a. Complete cross-allergenicity between different cephalosporins should be assumed.
         b. Partial cross-allergenicity occurs between penicillins and cephalosporins.
       2. Other effects include nausea and diarrhea and opportunistic infections; some cephalosporins (eg, cefotetan) cause hypoprothrombinemia and disulfiram-like reactions with ethanol.
    D. Carbapenems
       1. Imipenem and **meropenem** are bactericidal, penicillinase-resistant antibiotics with wide activity against gram-positive and gram-negative bacteria including anaerobes.
       2. Carbapenems are intravenous agents eliminated by the kidney (reduce the dose in renal dysfunction); imipenem is used with cilastatin, which blocks its metabolism by renal dihydropeptidases.
       3. Toxicities include nausea, diarrhea, skin rash, and seizures at high doses.

E. **Vancomycin**
1. **Mechanisms:** Vancomycin is a bactericidal inhibitor of cell wall synthesis.
   a. It inhibits glycosylation reactions by binding to the D-Ala-D-Ala terminal of the pentapeptide chains of peptidoglycans.
   b. Resistance (in enterococci) involves decreased binding of the drug via replacement of the terminal D-Ala by D-lactate.
2. **Pharmacokinetics:** Vancomycin is not absorbed from the gastrointestinal tract; given parenterally it penetrates most tissues and undergoes renal elimination (reduce the dose in renal dysfunction).
3. **Clinical uses:** Vancomycin is the drug of choice for methicillin-resistant *Staphylococcus aureus* (MRSA) and a back-up drug for enterococcal infections and for pseudomembranous colitis.
4. **Toxicities** include chills, fevers, diffuse flushing, potential ototoxicity, and nephrotoxicity.

PNEUMOCOCCAL RESISTANCE TO ANTIBIOTICS

CLINICAL
CORRELATION

- *In the past decade drug-resistant Streptococcus pneumoniae (DRSP) strains have become increasingly prevalent worldwide.*
- *Resistance to the penicillins confers decreased susceptibility to most other β-lactam antibiotics, the mechanism involving changes in penicillin-binding proteins.*
- *DRSP strains are commonly resistant to macrolides, tetracyclines, and trimethoprim-sulfamethoxazole, but presently respond to newer fluoroquinolones including levofloxacin and sparfloxacin.*
- *Vancomycin remains active against most pneumococci.*

III. **Inhibitors of Protein Synthesis: Macrolides, Clindamycin, Tetracyclines, and Chloramphenicol**

A. **Mechanisms of Action & Resistance**
1. Although of diverse chemical structures, all of these drugs are bacteriostatic inhibitors of protein synthesis acting at the ribosomal level (Figure 7–2).
2. **Mechanisms of action: Macrolides** and **clindamycin** bind to the 50S subunit to block translocation; **chloramphenicol** also binds to the 50S subunit, but inhibits transpeptidation by preventing binding of the aminoacyl moiety of charged tRNA; **tetracyclines** bind to the 30S subunit to prevent binding of the charged tRNA to the acceptor site of the ribosomal–mRNA complex.
3. **Mechanisms of resistance:** In gram-positive cocci, resistance to macrolides involves methylation of the 50S "receptor," preventing binding of the antibiotics. Resistance to chloramphenicol involves formation of acetyltransferases that inactivate the drug. Decreased intracellular accumulation is the primary mechanism of resistance to tetracyclines.

B. **Macrolide Antibiotics**
1. **Drugs** include **erythromycin, azithromycin,** and **clarithromycin.**
2. **Pharmacokinetics:** All drugs have good oral bioavailability.
   a. Erythromycin (biliary excretion) and clarithromycin (metabolism and renal clearance) have half-lives of less than 5 hours.
   b. Azithromycin accumulates in tissues and undergoes renal elimination with a half-life of more than 3 days; a single dose is adequate for management of nongonococcal urethritis.

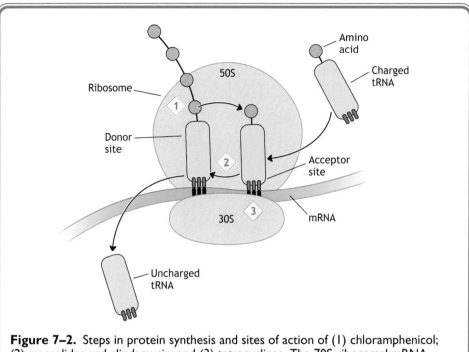

Figure 7–2. Steps in protein synthesis and sites of action of (1) chloramphenicol; (2) macrolides and clindamycin; and (3) tetracyclines. The 70S ribosomal mRNA complex is shown with its 50S and 30S subunits. The peptidyl-tRNA at the donor site donates the growing peptide chain to the aminoacyl-tRNA at the acceptor site in a reaction catalyzed by peptidyltransferase. Discharged of its peptide, the tRNA is released from the donor site to make way for translocation of the newly formed peptidyl-tRNA. The acceptor site is then free to be occupied by the next charged aminoacyl-tRNA. See text for additional details. (Reproduced, with permission, from Katzung BG [editor]: *Basic & Clinical Pharmacology,* 9th ed. McGraw-Hill, 2004.)

3. **Clinical uses:** Macrolides are used for infections caused by gram-positive cocci (not MRSA, and some pneumococcal strains are also resistant), *Mycoplasma pneumoniae,* chlamydial species, *Ureaplasma urealyticum,* and *Legionella pneumophila.*

   a. Azithromycin is also active against *Haemophilus influenzae* and *Moraxella catarrhalis.*

   b. Clarithromycin is active against *Helicobacter pylori.*

4. **Toxicities:** Erythromycin causes gastrointestinal distress and its estolate form may cause cholestasis (avoid in pregnancy). Both erythromycin and clarithromycin inhibit cytochrome P-450s and may enhance the effects of other drugs including carbamazepine, theophylline, and warfarin. Azithromycin does not inhibit drug metabolism and is safe in pregnancy.

C. **Clindamycin**

1. **Pharmacokinetics:** Clindamycin is effective orally, with good tissue penetration. It is eliminated by metabolism, biliary secretion, and renal clearance.

2. **Clinical uses:** Clindamycin is active versus gram-positive cocci (not MRSA) and anaerobes including *Bacteroides* strains. It is prophylactic against enterococcal endocarditis in penicillin-allergic patients and is a back-up drug for infections caused by *Pneumocystis carinii* and *Toxoplasma gondii*.

3. **Toxicities** include gastrointestinal distress, skin rash, and opportunistic infections including pseudomembranous colitis.

D. **Tetracyclines**

1. **Drugs** include **tetracycline** and **doxycycline.**
2. **Pharmacokinetics:** Tetracyclines have good oral bioavailability (avoid antacids) with wide tissue penetration; most are eliminated via the kidney, but a large fraction of doxycycline appears in the feces.
3. **Clinical uses:** These drugs are used to treat infections due to *Mycoplasma pneumoniae*, chlamydial species, *Rickettsia*, and *Vibrio*.
   a. Tetracyclines are back-up drugs in syphilis and are used prophylactically in chronic bronchitis and acne.
   b. Tetracycline is used against *Helicobacter pylori*.
   c. Doxycycline is the drug of choice in Lyme disease.
   d. Demeclocycline is used in management of the syndrome of inappropriate secretion of antidiuretic hormone (SIADH).
4. **Toxicities:** Tetracyclines cause gastrointestinal disturbances, opportunistic infections, tooth enamel dysplasia, and bone growth irregularities in children, as well as phototoxicity, and dizziness.
   a. Although rare, hepatic dysfunction has occurred in overdose.
   b. Outdated tetracyclines may cause nephrotoxicity (Fanconi's syndrome).

E. **Chloramphenicol**

1. **Pharmacokinetics:** Chloramphenicol is orally effective with wide tissue penetration. It is metabolized by glucuronosyltransferase (this enzyme may be deficient in neonates).
2. **Clinical uses:** Chloramphenicol is currently a back-up drug in bacterial meningitis, typhoid fever, rickettsial diseases, and *Bacteroides* infections.
3. **Toxicities** include nausea and diarrhea, opportunistic infections, bone marrow suppression (dose dependent and reversible), and aplastic anemia (very rare). The "gray baby" syndrome, characterized by cyanosis and cardiovascular collapse, occurred in neonates with inadequate glucuronosyltransferase.

IV. **Inhibitors of Protein Synthesis: Aminoglycosides, Streptogramins, and Linezolid**

A. **Mechanisms of Action & Resistance**

1. **Mechanism of action:** Aminoglycosides are bactericidal inhibitors of protein synthesis.
   a. Intracellular accumulation is oxygen-dependent—anaerobes are innately resistant.
   b. By binding to the 30S ribosomal subunit, aminoglycosides block formation of the initiation complex, prevent translocation, and cause misreading of mRNA (Figure 7–3).
   c. Streptogramins are also bactericidal, binding to a site on the 50S subunit and blocking extrusion of nascent polypeptides; they also inhibit tRNA synthetase.
   d. Linezolid (bacteriostatic) also binds to a 50S subunit site to block initiation.

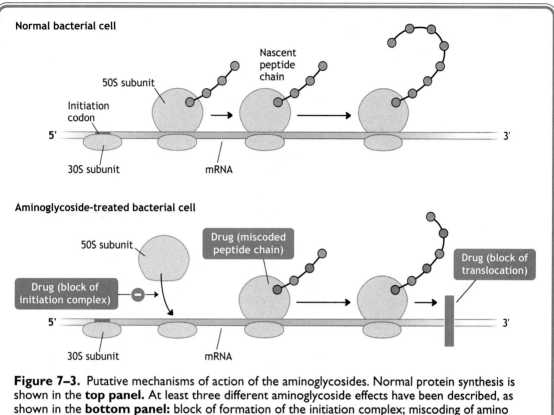

Figure 7–3. Putative mechanisms of action of the aminoglycosides. Normal protein synthesis is shown in the **top panel.** At least three different aminoglycoside effects have been described, as shown in the **bottom panel:** block of formation of the initiation complex; miscoding of amino acids in the emerging peptide chain due to misreading of the mRNA; and block of translocation on mRNA. Block of movement of the ribosome may occur after the formation of a single initiation complex, resulting in an mRNA chain with only a single ribosome on it, a so-called monosome.

    2. Mechanisms of resistance: Resistance to aminoglycosides is common in gram-positive bacteria, occurring via plasmid-mediated formation of inactivating transferases. Streptogramins and linezolid are new antibiotics and resistance patterns are undetermined.

  B. Pharmacokinetics of Aminoglycosides

    1. Absorption and distribution: As polar compounds these drugs are not absorbed orally or widely distributed. Parenteral administration is required for systemic and most tissue infections.

    2. Elimination: Renal clearance of all aminoglycosides is proportional to glomerular filtration rate (GFR) and major dose reductions are needed in renal dysfunction. Elimination half-lives are 2–3 hours.

ONCE-DAILY DOSING OF AMINOGLYCOSIDES

• *Despite their short half-lives, the administration of aminoglycosides once daily is as effective as conventional dosing regimens and results in less nephrotoxicity.*

- A **postantibiotic effect** *(PAE) occurs, in which killing action continues when plasma levels have fallen below expected minimal inhibitory concentrations.*
- *Aminoglycosides cause a concentration-dependent, rather than a time-dependent killing action, but nephrotoxicity appears to be dependent on both dosage and time.*

    C. **Clinical Uses of Aminoglycosides**
       1. **Gentamicin, tobramycin, and amikacin:** Aminoglycosides are commonly used for infections caused by aerobic gram-negative bacilli, including *Escherichia coli* and species of *Enterobacter, Klebsiella, Proteus, Pseudomonas,* and *Serratia.* Synergism occurs with penicillins against enterococci and *Pseudomonas* strains.
       2. **Streptomycin and neomycin:** Streptomycin is used in regimens for tuberculosis and in cholera and tularemia. Due to its toxicity neomycin is used only by topical application.

    D. **Toxicities of Aminoglycosides**
       1. **Nephrotoxicity** usually involves acute tubular necrosis, with an incidence of 6–7%. Once-daily dosing reduces toxic effects on the kidney.
       2. **Ototoxicity** may involve auditory or vestibular dysfunction, with an incidence of 2–3%, which may not be fully reversible.
       3. **Contact dermatitis** is especially frequent with neomycin.

    E. **Streptogramins & Linezolid**
       1. **Drugs:** The streptogramin combination of **quinupristin** and **dalfopristin** is used intravenously for treatment of infections caused by MRSA, and for both vancomycin-resistant *Staphylococcus aureus* (VRSA) and vancomycin-resistant enterococcus (VRE).
          a. Linezolid has similar clinical indications and is also active against penicillin-resistant pneumococci.
          b. Currently there is no cross-resistance with other inhibitors of protein synthesis.
       2. **Toxicities:** Streptogramins cause arthralgia and myalgia; they are potent inhibitors of cytochrome P-450s involved in drug metabolism.

  V. Inhibitors of Folic Acid Synthesis: Sulfonamides and Trimethoprim
    A. **Mechanisms of Action**
       1. **Sulfonamides:** These drugs are structurally similar to *para*-aminobenzoic acid (PABA), a precursor used by microorganisms in the synthesis of folates. Sulfonamides inhibit dihydropteroate synthase, the first step in folic acid synthesis (Figure 7–4).
       2. **Trimethoprim:** A structural analog of dihydrofolic acid, trimethoprim inhibits the dihydrofolate reductase (DHFR) in bacteria. Pyrimethamine, another antifol, inhibits DHFR in protozoans.
       3. **Sequential blockade:** The combination of sulfamethoxazole and trimethoprim causes a sequential blockade of folic acid synthesis and results in antibacterial synergy.

    B. **Mechanism of Resistance**
       1. **Sulfonamides:** Mechanisms include changed sensitivity of dihydropteroate synthase, increased production of PABA, and decreased intracellular accumulation of the drugs.
       2. **Trimethoprim:** Resistance involves a change in sensitivity of DHFR.

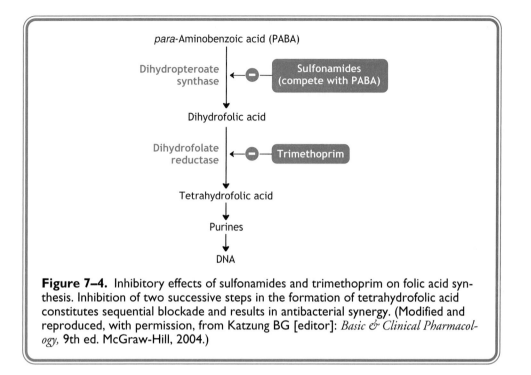

para-Aminobenzoic acid (PABA)

Dihydropteroate synthase ← ⊖ — Sulfonamides (compete with PABA)

Dihydrofolic acid

Dihydrofolate reductase ← ⊖ — Trimethoprim

Tetrahydrofolic acid

Purines

DNA

Figure 7–4. Inhibitory effects of sulfonamides and trimethoprim on folic acid synthesis. Inhibition of two successive steps in the formation of tetrahydrofolic acid constitutes sequential blockade and results in antibacterial synergy. (Modified and reproduced, with permission, from Katzung BG [editor]: *Basic & Clinical Pharmacology,* 9th ed. McGraw-Hill, 2004.)

C. Pharmacokinetics

1. Most sulfonamides are effective orally.

a. Intact drugs or acetylated metabolites are eliminated via the kidney, but may cause crystalluria in acidic urine.

b. Sulfonamides bind to plasma proteins and can displace other bound drugs (eg, phenytoin and warfarin) and bilirubin.

2. Trimethoprim is well absorbed orally and penetrates tissues effectively. Trimethoprim is eliminated largely unchanged by the kidney.

D. Clinical Uses

1. As individual drugs sulfonamides may be used for simple urinary tract infections (UTIs) (eg, sulfisoxazole), for ocular chlamydial infections (sulfacetamide), in burn dressings, and for ulcerative colitis (sulfasalazine).

2. Trimethoprim-sulfamethoxazole (TMP-SMX) is effective in many UTIs and in respiratory, ear, and sinus infections including those due to *Haemophilus influenzae* and *Moraxella catarrhalis.* It is the drug of choice for prevention and treatment of *Pneumocystis carinii* pneumonia.

E. Toxicities

1. Sulfonamides: Adverse effects include hypersensitivity reactions (incidence of 4–6%), nausea and diarrhea, hemolysis in glucose-6-phosphate dehydrogenase (G6PD) deficiency, phototoxicity, crystalluria, and drug interactions.

2. TMP-SMX: Adverse effects include those of sulfonamides plus hematotoxicity (anemia and granulocytopenia), especially in malnourished or immunodeficient patients.

METHICILLIN-RESISTANT *STAPHYLOCOCCUS AUREUS*

- *MRSA strains are resistant to all β-lactam antibiotics.*
- *They are also usually resistant to macrolide antibiotics, older fluoroquinolones, and trimethoprim-sulfamethoxazole.*
- *Vancomycin presently has activity against most strains of MRSA, but resistance is increasing.*
- *Alternative drugs for MRSA include quinupristin-dalfopristin and linezolid.*

VI. Inhibitors of Nucleic Acid Synthesis: Fluoroquinolones

A. Concepts

1. **Fluoroquinolones** are derivatives of nalidixic acid.
2. **Norfloxacin** and **ciprofloxacin** are prototypes, the latter being used so extensively during the past decade that resistance is becoming problematic.
3. Newer fluoroquinolones may have activities against specific organisms; they may also exhibit distinctive toxicities.

B. Mechanisms of Action and Resistance

1. **Mechanisms of action:** Fluoroquinolones are bactericidal inhibitors of nucleic acid synthesis. They inhibit both topoisomerase II (DNA gyrase), blocking relaxation of supercoiled DNA, and topoisomerase IV, preventing separation of the replicated DNA.
2. **Mechanisms of resistance:** Resistance is increasing, especially in gram-positive cocci. Mechanisms include decreased intracellular accumulation of drug and changes in sensitivity to inhibition of the topisomerases.

C. Pharmacokinetics

1. Antacids may interfere with oral bioavailability.
2. Renal clearance is via active tubular secretion; dose reductions are needed in renal dysfunction. Fluoroquinolones have short half-lives.

D. Clinical Uses

1. **General:** Fluoroquinolones have a wide spectrum of activity that includes most bacteria associated with genitourinary, gastrointestinal, and upper respiratory tract infections.
2. **Specific: Ciprofloxacin** and **ofloxacin** are used in single doses for gonorrhea, but resistance is increasing. **Levofloxacin** and **sparfloxacin,** with activity against *Mycoplasma pneumoniae* and PRSP, are used in community-acquired pneumonia. **Moxifloxacin** and **trovafloxacin** are newer drugs with broad activity that includes drug-resistant pneumococci, *Mycoplasma pneumoniae,* anaerobes, and *Chlamydia.*

E. Toxicities

1. Adverse effects common to all fluoroquinolones include gastrointestinal distress, skin rash, tendinitis, headache, and dizziness.
   a. Seizures have occurred in overdose and in susceptible patients.
   b. Fluoroquinolones are not recommended for use in pregnancy and small children, since animal studies show effects on collagen metabolism.
2. Phototoxicity has occurred with fluoroquinolones (eg, sparfloxacin) and the drugs have been reported to prolong the QT interval in susceptible patients. Trovafloxacin has hepatotoxic potential.

VII. Antimycobacterial Drugs

A. Concepts

1. **Drug combinations:** Chemotherapy of tuberculosis involves drug combinations to delay the development of resistance and to enhance activity. In many cases directly observed therapy (DOT) is necessary to ensure patient compliance.

2. **Major drugs:** Standard drugs used in tuberculosis include **isoniazid, rifampin, ethambutol, pyrazinamide,** and **streptomycin.** Fluoroquinolones and also several older antitubercular drugs may be used in regimens for management of multidrug-resistant infections.

3. **Prophylaxis:** Isoniazid and rifampin are used for latent tuberculosis infection.

B. Isoniazid (INH)

1. **Mechanisms of action and resistance:** INH is converted by mycobacterial catalase to a metabolite that inhibits mycolic acid synthesis.
   a. High-level resistance involves deletions in the *kat*G gene that codes for catalase.
   b. Low-level resistance involves deletions in the *inh*A gene that codes for the target acyl carrier protein.

2. **Pharmacokinetics:** INH is metabolized by *N*-acetyltransferase. Genotypic variability exists, with fast acetylators needing high doses of INH.

3. **Toxicities** include neurotoxicity (offset by vitamin B_6), hepatitis (age dependent), hemolysis in G6PD deficiency, and rare lupuslike reactions.

C. Rifampin

1. **Mechanisms of action and resistance:** Rifampin inhibits DNA-dependent RNA polymerase. Resistance occurs via changes in polymerase sensitivity to inhibition.

2. **Pharmacokinetics:** Rifampin undergoes hepatic metabolism to red-orange-colored metabolites.

3. **Toxicities:** Light-chain proteinuria, gastrointestinal distress, and rash are most common.
   a. A flulike syndrome may occur at high doses.
   b. Rifampin induces drug-metabolizing enzymes and may decrease the effectiveness of other drugs including anticonvulsants, contraceptive steroids, and warfarin.

D. Ethambutol & Pyrazinamide

1. **Ethambutol** inhibits the synthesis of arabinogalactan, a component of mycobacterial cell walls. Its most distinctive toxicity is dose-dependent and reversible retrobulbar neuritis.

2. **Pyrazinamide** requires bioactivation for activity, but its precise target is undetermined. There is minimal cross-resistance with other agents and the drug may be valuable in short-course treatment regimens. Toxicities include polyarthralgia, hyperuricemia, phototoxicity, and exacerbation of porphyria.

E. Drugs for *Mycobacterium avium-intracellulare* Infection

1. Prophylaxis involves azithromycin or clarithromycin.

2. Treatment involves clarithromycin plus ethambutol with or without rifampin or rifabutin.

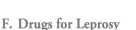

F. Drugs for Leprosy

1. **Dapsone,** the most active drug against *Mycobacterium leprae,* is also a back-up drug for *Pneumocystis carinii* pneumonia. Toxicities include gastrointestinal irritation, skin rash, methemoglobinemia, and hemolysis in G6PD deficiency.

2. Alternative drugs are rifampin or clofazimine, which are used in resistance or dapsone intolerance.

ANTIBIOTICS TO BE AVOIDED IN PREGNANCY

- *Aminoglycosides* have caused ototoxicity in the developing fetus.
- *Clarithromycin* is embryotoxic, based on results of animal studies.
- *Erythromycin estolate* increases the incidence of cholestasis in the pregnant patient.
- *Fluoroquinolones* have deleterious effects on collagen metabolism in animals.
- *Tetracyclines* interfere with bone and tooth formation via calcium chelation.
- *Sulfonamides* (used in the third trimester) may displace bilirubin from plasma proteins in the fetus and neonate, causing kernicterus.
- *Metronidazole* is mutagenic in the Ames test.

VIII. Miscellaneous Antimicrobials

A. Metronidazole

1. **Mechanism of action: Metronidazole** undergoes reductive metabolism in anaerobes, forming a metabolite that interferes with nucleic acid synthesis.

2. **Clinical uses:** Metronidazole is the drug of choice in amebiasis, giardiasis, and trichomoniasis, and in infections caused by *Bacteroides fragilis, Clostridium difficile,* and *Gardnerella vaginalis;* it is also used in the eradication of *Helicobacter pylori.*

3. **Toxicities:** Gastrointestinal irritation, headache, dizziness, and dark-colored urine are common. Disulfiramlike reactions occur with ethanol.

B. Fosfomycin

1. **Mechanism of action and resistance: Fosfomycin** inhibits enolpyruvate transferase, preventing formation of *N*-acetylmuramic acid needed for bacterial cell wall synthesis. Resistance occurs via decreased intracellular accumulation.

2. **Clinical use:** Fosfomycin is used to treat UTIs.

C. Urinary Antiseptics

1. Oral administration of **nitrofurantoin** results in urinary levels adequate for eradication of most urinary pathogens except *Proteus* and *Pseudomonas* species. Toxicities include gastrointestinal distress, skin rash, phototoxicity, and hemolysis in G6PD deficiency.

2. **Nalidixic acid** is a quinolone with antibacterial activity similar to that of nitrofurantoin. Toxicities include glycosuria, skin rash, phototoxicity, and ocular dysfunction.

3. **Methenamine** is a urinary acidifier that releases formaldehyde below pH 5.5. Insoluble complexes form if methenamine is used with sulfonamides.

D. Disinfectants & Antiseptics

1. **Acids, alcohols,** and **aldehydes** include ethanol (70%), formaldehyde, acetic acid, and salicylic acid.

2. Halogens include iodine and hypochlorous acid.
  a. Halazone is used in water purification.
  b. Sodium hypochlorite (in household bleach) is used for disinfection of blood spills that may contain human immunodeficiency virus or hepatitis B virus.
3. Oxidizing agents include hydrogen peroxide and potassium permanganate.
4. Heavy metals include merbromin and silver sulfadiazine.
5. Chlorinated phenols include hexachlorophene and chlorhexidine, which are widely used in surgical scrub routines. Lindane is used for mite or lice infestation.
6. Cationic surfactants include benzalkonium chloride and cetylpyridinium chloride, which have been used for disinfection of surgical instruments, but may foster growth of resistant gram-negative bacteria.

ANTIBACTERIAL DRUGS AND PHOTOTOXICITY

- *Many systemic drugs cause phototoxicity reactions involving delayed erythema and edema, followed by skin hyperpigmentation and desquamation.*
- *Fluoroquinolones, sulfonamides, and tetracyclines often cause such reactions, localized mainly to regions of the body exposed to ultraviolet light.*
- *Other antimicrobial drugs that cause phototoxicity include griseofulvin, lincomycin, nalidixic acid, pyrazinamide, and trimethoprim.*

CLINICAL PROBLEMS

A patient with no apparent comorbid condition exhibits symptoms of a community-acquired pneumonia with fever, chest pain, rales on chest auscultation, and purulent sputum. There are no extrapulmonary manifestations. A chest x-ray confirms the presence of an infiltrate. Samples of blood and sputum are sent for microbiological analysis.

1. Concern is expressed about the possibility that the infection in this patient may be caused by drug-resistant pneumococci. Consequently, empiric treatment should involve the administration of which of the following?

   A. Amoxicillin

   B. Erythromycin

   C. Levofloxacin

   D. Metronidazole

   E. Penicillin G

2. If the patient had a nonproductive cough, no chest pain, and extrapulmonary manifestations of disease including diarrhea, mental confusion, and a rash, the antibiotic chosen for treatment should have activity against which of the following?

   A. Enterococci

   B. *Giardia* species

   C. *Haemophilus influenzae*

D. *Mycoplasma pneumoniae*

E. Respiratory viruses

A 22-year-old male presents with dysuria, pruritus, and a milky penile discharge. Examination of a postmicturition urethral swab reveals gram-negative cocci and further microbiological analysis is pursued. At this point the patient is treated with a single intramuscular injection of ceftriaxone and a single oral dose of azithromycin.

3. If this patient had an established hypersensitivity to β-lactam antibiotics, which one of the following drugs is most likely to be effective and safe in the treatment of urethral gonorrhea if it is administered in a single dose?

   A. Amoxicillin

   B. Ciprofloxacin

   C. Doxycycline

   D. Gentamicin

   E. Vancomycin

4. Azithromycin provides coverage for nongonococcal pathogens that are often associated with gonococcal urethritis, but the drug has no activity against which of the following?

   A. Any of the following organisms

   B. Chlamydial species

   C. Mycoplasmal species

   D. *Trichomonas vaginalis*

   E. *Ureaplasma urealyticum*

Factors that predispose to staphylococcal infections include diabetes, indwelling intravenous catheters, neutropenia, and intravenous drug abuse. If left untreated, staphylococcal bacteremia has an 80% mortality rate.

5. In a patient with bacteremia due to a catalase-positive coagulase-positive staphylococcal species, which of the following antibiotics is least likely to be effective?

   A. Amoxicillin

   B. Cephalexin

   C. Clindamycin

   D. Erythromycin

   E. Nafcillin

6. In the case of a staphylococcal bacteremia due to a methicillin-resistant *Staphylococcus aureus* (MRSA), which of the following drugs is most likely to be effective?

   A. Amoxicillin-clavulanate

   B. Ceftriaxone

   C. Erythromycin

   D. Tetracycline

   E. Vancomycin

A 35-year-old female patient presents with symptoms that include a productive cough, fever, night sweats, and weight loss. Sputum is submitted for smear, culture, and susceptibility testing. The sputum smear is positive for acid-fast bacilli and a chest x-ray reveals upper lobe patchy infiltrates. Laboratory tests requested include complete blood count, liver function enzymes, bilirubin, creatinine, and uric acid. The patient is hospitalized and is to remain in isolation during treatment until the sputum becomes smear-negative.

7. Regarding the empiric treatment of pulmonary tuberculosis contracted in communities in which INH resistance is greater than 4%, which of the following statements is accurate?

   A. All patients with pulmonary tuberculosis must undergo antibiotic treatment for at least 18 months

   B. Combination drug treatment initially with four antitubercular drugs is anticipated

   C. Isoniazid is not used in antitubercular drug regimens if the resistance rate in the community is more than 4%

   D. Patients should have baseline audiometric testing prior to drug treatment

   E. Potential drug interactions necessitate discontinuance of all drugs taken by the patient for other clinical conditions

8. Which of the following matched pairs of drug: adverse effect is accurate?

   A. Ethambutol: hepatitis

   B. Isoniazid: decreased visual acuity and color discrimination defects

   C. Pyrazinamide: hyperuricemia

   D. Rifampin: ototoxicity

   E. Streptomycin: induction of hepatic drug-metabolizing enzymes

ANSWERS

1. The answer is C. Bacteria (especially pneumococci) are responsible for many cases of community-acquired pneumonia. Pneumococci are gaining resistance not only to β-lactams, but also to macrolide antibiotics. Drug-resistant streptococci are susceptible to levofloxacin, sparfloxacin, moxifloxacin, linezolid, and vancomycin.

2. The answer is D. *Mycoplasma pneumoniae, Chlamydia pneumoniae,* and *Legionella pneumophila* are responsible for approximately 15% of community-acquired pneumonia cases. A nonproductive cough, absence of chest pain, and extrapulmonary symptoms are diagnostic features. Even in the absence of such symptoms antibiotic coverage against these organisms should be provided in the treatment of a community-acquired pneumonia.

3. The answer is B. Ciprofloxacin and ofloxacin are usually effective in single oral doses for treatment of gonorrhea. Spectinomycin (intramuscularly) is also usually effective in

a single dose. None of these drugs is effective (in single doses) against accompanying nongonococcal pathogens in gonococcal urethritis. Tetracyclines are effective against both gonococci and "atypicals" but not in single doses.

4. The answer is D. Three of the organisms listed, together with herpes simplex virus, are contributory pathogens in gonococcal urethritis. Chlamydial, mycoplasmal, and ureaplasmal species are responsive to treatment with macrolide antibiotics (eg, azithromycin) and tetracyclines, but infections due to *Trichomonas vaginalis* should be treated with metronidazole.

5. The answer is A. Most strains of coagulase-positive staphylococci produce β-lactamases that inactivate penicillins, including amoxicillin and ampicillin, unless they are used in conjunction with penicillinase inhibitors such as clavulanic acid and sulbactam. Penicillinase-resistant penicillins (eg, nafcillin) are effective in most staphylococcal infections, as are many other antibiotics including cephalosporins and macrolides.

6. The answer is E. No β-lactam antibiotics, macrolides, or tetracyclines are effective against methicillin-resistant staphylococci. The drug of choice for infections caused by such organisms is vancomycin. Linezolid and the streptogramins are also effective.

7. The answer is B. An empiric four-drug regimen that includes isoniazid, rifampin, pyrazinamide, and either ethambutol or streptomycin is used in pulmonary tuberculosis for which the INH resistance rate exceeds 4%. After 2 months, if the isolate proves to be fully drug-susceptible, a two-drug regimen of isoniazid and rifampin is continued for a further 4 months ("short-course" therapy).

8. The answer is C. The antitubercular drug most associated with hepatitis is isoniazid. Ethambutol causes dose-dependent and reversible ocular dysfunction. Aminoglycosides (eg, streptomycin) cause ototoxicity and nephrotoxicity. Rifampin, an inducer of hepatic drug-metabolizing enzymes, is involved in many drug interactions.

CHAPTER 8
ANTIFUNGAL, ANTIVIRAL, AND ANTIPARASITIC DRUGS

I. Antifungal Drugs

A. Concepts

1. The polyene **amphotericin B** and azoles (**fluconazole** and **itraconazole**) are the major drugs used in systemic mycoses.
2. They are selectively toxic to fungi because they interact with, or block the synthesis of, ergosterol, an essential component of fungal cell membranes.
3. Figure 8–1 depicts the actions of these and other antifungal agents.

B. Amphotericin B & Nystatin

1. **Mechanisms of action and resistance:** Polyene antifungals bind to ergosterol, forming artificial pores that increase membrane permeability. Resistance, though rare, occurs via a decreased level, or structural change in, membrane sterols.
2. **Pharmacokinetics:** Amphotericin B (Amp B), which is given by slow intravenous infusion, penetrates weakly into the central nervous system (CNS).
    a. Renal elimination predominates and the drug has a long half-life.
    b. **Nystatin** is too toxic for systemic use and is applied locally.
3. **Clinical uses:** Amp B is a drug of choice for aspergillosis, systemic candidiasis, cryptococcal infections, histoplasmosis, mucormycosis, and sporotrichosis. Nystatin is used by topical application (eg, treatment of oral or vaginal candidiasis).
4. **Toxicities:**
    a. AMB causes infusion-related effects including hypotension, chills, fevers, and rigor.
    b. Analgesics, antihistamines, and steroids may be used supportively.
    c. Nephrotoxicity of Amp B is dose limiting, resulting in tubular acidosis, electrolyte imbalance, and anemia.
    d. Full hydration of patients and the use of liposomal forms of Amp B reduce nephrotoxicity.

C. Azole Antifungals

1. **Mechanisms of action and resistance:** Azoles interfere with cell membrane synthesis by inhibiting a fungal cytochrome P-450 (CYP450) that converts lanosterol to ergosterol; resistance occurs via a change in sensitivity of this target enzyme or decreased intracellular accumulation.
2. **Pharmacokinetics:** Azoles have good oral efficacy, but absorption may be inhibited by antacids.

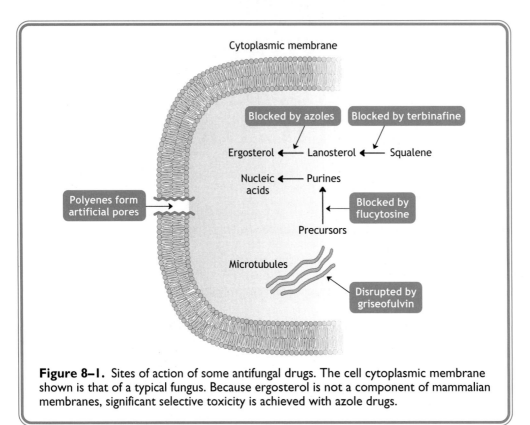

Figure 8–1. Sites of action of some antifungal drugs. The cell cytoplasmic membrane shown is that of a typical fungus. Because ergosterol is not a component of mammalian membranes, significant selective toxicity is achieved with azole drugs.

    a. Fluconazole is the only azole that effectively enters the CSF.
    b. Ketoconazole, itraconazole, and **voriconazole** are metabolized in the liver; fluconazole is eliminated via the kidney.
  3. Clinical uses: Clinical uses vary.
    a. Ketoconazole is used for mucocutaneous candidiasis and dermatophytoses.
    b. Fluconazole is a drug of choice in esophageal candidiasis, candidemia, and coccidial infections; it is also active in cryptococcal meningitis.
    c. Itraconazole has the widest spectrum of the azoles and is a drug of choice in blastomycosis and sporotrichosis.
    d. Voriconazole is used for treatment of invasive aspergillosis.
    e. Clotrimazole and miconazole are topical antifungal agents.
  4. Toxicities: Azoles cause a variety of adverse effects.
    a. Gastrointestinal distress is the most common side effect.
    b. Azoles (especially ketoconazole) may cause endocrine dysfunction via inhibition of CYP450s involved in synthesis of cortisol and testosterone.
    c. Hepatic drug-metabolizing CYP450s are inhibited by azoles, especially ketoconazole.
    d. Voriconazole use is associated with visual and hepatic dysfunction; the drug is contraindicated in pregnancy.

D. **Flucytosine**
1. **Mechanisms of action and resistance:** Flucytosine (5-FC) is accumulated in fungi via a permease and converted by cytosine deaminase to 5-fluorouracil (5-FU), an inhibitor of thymidylate synthase. Resistance occurs rapidly in fungi deficient in these enzymes.
2. **Pharmacokinetics:** 5-FC is orally active and penetrates most tissues including the CNS. It is eliminated via the kidney; dose reduction is needed in renal dysfunction.
3. **Clinical uses:** 5-FC is used in combination with Amp B in candidemia or cryptococcal meningitis.
4. **Toxicities:** 5-FC causes bone marrow suppression.

E. **Griseofulvin**
1. **Mechanisms of action and resistance:** Griseofulvin disrupts microtubular functions in dermatophytes and may inhibit nucleic acid synthesis; resistant strains do not accumulate the drug.
2. **Pharmacokinetics:** Orally active, griseofulvin accumulates in keratin and is eliminated via the bile.
3. **Clinical uses:** Griseofulvin is used for dermatophytoses of the skin, hair, and nails.
4. **Toxicities:** Adverse effects include gastrointestinal irritation, headaches, and phototoxicity. Griseofulvin decreases the bioavailability of warfarin and causes a disulfiramlike effect with ethanol.

F. **Terbinafine**
1. **Mechanism of action:** Terbinafine inhibits squalene epoxidase, causing high levels of squalene, which inhibit ergosterol synthesis.
2. **Pharmacokinetics:** Terbinafine is orally active and accumulates in keratin.
3. **Clinical uses:** Terbinafine is used for dermatophytoses of the skin, hair, and nails.
4. **Toxicities:** Adverse effects include gastrointestinal irritation, skin rash, headaches, and elevation of liver function enzymes.

G. **Caspofungin**
1. **Mechanism of action:** Inhibits the synthesis of β(1-2)glycan, a critical component of fungal cell walls.
2. **Clinical uses and toxicity:** Used intravenously for management of invasive aspergillosis and systemic candidiasis. Adverse effects include mild infusion-related reactions and headache.

ANTIFUNGAL DRUG INTERACTIONS

- *Ketoconazole and related drugs inhibit CYP450-mediated metabolism of cyclosporine, didanosine, lovastatin, phenytoin, quinidine, verapamil, and warfarin.*
- *Oral absorption of azoles may be impeded by proton pump inhibitors (eg, omeprazole), H_2-receptor blockers (eg, ranitidine), and other antacids.*
- *Griseofulvin increases the metabolism of warfarin.*

II. Antiviral Drugs

A. **Concepts**
1. Antiviral drugs act at several stages of viral replication, but most drugs inhibit nucleic acid or late protein synthesis (Figure 8–2).

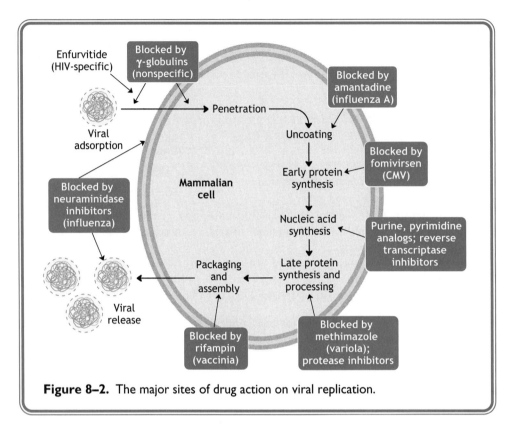

Figure 8–2. The major sites of drug action on viral replication.

2. Many antiviral drugs are antimetabolites that resemble naturally occurring compounds.
3. Some drugs require phosphorylation by viral or host cell kinases prior to exerting their antiviral actions.

B. **Acyclovir**
   1. **Mechanism of action:** Acyclovir is monophosphorylated by viral **thymidine kinase** and further phosphorylated by host kinases to the nucleotide; this is a substrate and inhibitor of viral DNA polymerase, and when incorporated into DNA causes chain termination.
   2. **Mechanism of resistance:** Most resistant strains of herpes are deficient in thymidine kinase (TK⁻ strains); others have decreased sensitivity of DNA polymerase to inhibition.
   3. **Pharmacokinetics:** Acyclovir is orally active, but has a very short half-life requiring multiple daily doses.
      a. It is eliminated mainly by renal excretion.
      b. Topical and intravenous forms are available.
   4. **Clinical uses:** Acyclovir is used for treatment of mucocutaneous and genital herpes simplex virus (HSV), for prophylaxis in immunocompromised patients, and for varicella-zoster infections.
   5. **Toxicities:** Gastrointestinal distress and headache are common. Intravenous use may cause crystalluria, delirium, tremor, and seizures. Acyclovir is not hematotoxic.

6. **Newer anti-HSV drugs: Famciclovir** and **valacyclovir** have longer durations of action; they are not active against TK⁻ strains of HSV. **Penciclovir** is used topically.

ANTIMICROBIAL AND ANTIVIRAL PROPHYLAXIS

- *Acyclovir is effective in prophylaxis against recurrent genital herpes infections.*
- *Other nonsurgical prophylactic antimicrobial regimens with established efficacy include prevention of endocarditis (amoxicillin or ampicillin), recurrent otitis media (amoxicillin), rheumatic fever (penicillin G), and tuberculosis (isoniazid or rifampin).*
- *In AIDS patients, prophylactic regimens include trimethoprim-sulfamethoxazole against Pneumocystis carinii pneumonia and Toxoplasma encephalitis, and clarithromycin or rifabutin against Mycoplasma avium-intracellulare.*

C. **Ganciclovir**
   1. **Mechanisms of action and resistance:** Viral-specific enzymes (phosphotransferases) initiate bioactivation of ganciclovir and further phosphorylation occurs via host kinases.
      a. The nucleotide inhibits viral DNA polymerase, but does not cause chain termination.
      b. Resistance occurs via decreased viral phosphotransferases or changes in DNA polymerase.
   2. **Pharmacokinetics:** Ganciclovir is usually given intravenously. Intraocular implants can be used for cytomegalovirus (CMV) retinitis. Ganciclovir is eliminated by the kidney; the dose should be reduced in renal dysfunction.
   3. **Clinical uses:** Ganciclovir is used for prophylaxis and treatment of CMV infections.
   4. **Toxicities:** Adverse effects include hematotoxicity and neurotoxicity (seizures in overdose).

D. **Foscarnet**
   1. **Mechanisms of action and resistance:** Foscarnet inhibits viral RNA and DNA polymerases, but is not an antimetabolite (no bioactivation). Mutations in polymerase genes result in resistance.
   2. **Pharmacokinetics:** Foscarnet is administered intravenously; the drug undergoes renal elimination.
   3. **Clinical uses:** Foscarnet is used for prophylaxis and treatment of CMV infections and is active against ganciclovir-resistant CMV strains and TK⁻ strains of HSV.
   4. **Toxicities:** Adverse effects include nephrotoxicity, genitourinary ulceration, and neurotoxicity (seizures in overdose).

E. **Other Antiherpetic Drugs**
   1. **Cidofovir** is an antimetabolite that on bioactivation (nonviral) inhibits DNA polymerases of HSV, CMV, adenovirus, and papillomavirus. It is markedly nephrotoxic.
   2. **Vidarabine** is an antimetabolite active against HSV, varicella-zoster virus (VZV), and CMV. It is mainly used topically due to severe neuro- and hepatotoxicity.
   3. **Fomivirsen** is an antisense nucleotide that binds to mRNA of CMV, inhibiting early protein synthesis; it is injected intravitreally for CMV retinitis.

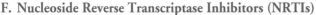

F. Nucleoside Reverse Transcriptase Inhibitors (NRTIs)

1. **Mechanisms of action and resistance:** NRTIs are phosphorylated by viral and host kinases to nucleotides that inhibit human immunodeficiency virus (HIV) reverse transcriptase and cause chain termination in viral DNA. Resistance is due to mutation at several sites of the *pol* gene that encodes reverse transcriptase.

2. **Drugs and pharmacokinetics: Zidovudine (ZDV)** is the prototype of a group that includes **didanosine (ddI), zalcitabine (ddC), lamivudine (3TC), stavudine (d4T),** and **abacavir.** Most NRTIs have good oral bioavailability and are eliminated via metabolism and/or renal elimination.

3. **Clinical uses:** NRTIs are standard components of anti-HIV drug regimens (usually two NRTIs plus a protease inhibitor).
   a. Zidovudine (with or without other anti-HIV drugs) is used as prophylaxis in needlestick accidents and to reduce vertical transmission in pregnancy.
   b. Lamivudine is also used with interferon-α or as an individual agent in hepatitis B infection.

4. **Toxicities:** Dose-limiting toxicities include bone marrow suppression (zidovudine), pancreatitis (didanosine), and peripheral neuropathy (zalcitabine and stavudine). Abacavir causes severe hypersensitivity reactions. NRTIs may cause lactic acidosis.

G. Nonnucleoside Reverse Transcriptase Inhibitors (NNRTIs)

1. **Mechanisms of action and resistance:** These drugs do not require metabolic activation, inhibiting viral RNA polymerases directly and allosterically.
   a. Resistance occurs rapidly if used as single agents (mutations in the reverse transcriptase gene).
   b. There is no cross-resistance with nucleoside inhibitors.

2. **Drugs and toxicities:** NNRTIs include **nevirapine** (severe hypersensitivity reactions), **delavirdine** (skin rash and teratogenicity), and **efavirenz** (neurotoxicity, hyperlipidemia, and teratogenicity).

H. Protease Inhibitors (PIs)

1. **Mechanisms of action and resistance:** These drugs inhibit aspartate protease, an enzyme that cleaves precursor proteins needed for producing mature virions of HIV. Resistance occurs via point mutations in the protease gene. Cross-resistance between PIs is incomplete.

2. **Clinical uses:** PIs are used in anti-HIV drug regimens that usually include two RTIs.

3. **Drugs and toxicities:** PIs include **indinavir** (hematotoxicity and nephrotoxicity), **ritonavir** (nausea, diarrhea, and inhibition of metabolism of many drugs including other PIs), **saquinavir** (neutropenia), **nelfinavir** (diarrhea and hypersensitivity), and **amprenavir** (hypersensitivity). Protease inhibitors may cause disorders of carbohydrate and lipid metabolism.

I. Enfurvitide

1. **Mechanism of action and resistance:** Enfurvitide is a synthetic peptide that binds to the gp41 subunit of the viral envelope protein, blocking fusion of the virus with cellular membranes. There is no cross-resistance with other anti-HIV drugs, but resistance may occur via mutations in the *env* gene.

2. **Clinical use and toxicity:** Enfurvitide is given subcutaneously with other anti-HIV agents in patients with persistent HIV replication despite ongoing therapy. Injection site reactions occur and an increased incidence of bacterial pneumonia has been reported.

Table 8–1. Miscellaneous antiviral drugs.

Drugs	Clinical Use	Mechanisms of Action	Toxicities
Amantadine	Influenza A	Prevents viral fusion and uncapping	Gastrointestinal distress, dizziness, slurred speech
Oseltamivir, zanamivir	Influenzas A and B	Inhibit neuraminidase and impede viral release	
Interferon-α	Hepatitis viruses (A, B, C), Kaposi's sarcoma, papillomatosis	Interferes with viral RNA and DNA synthesis	Neutropenia, fatigue, mental confusion, cardiomyopathy
Ribavirin	Respiratory syncitial virus, Hanta and Lassa viruses, hepatitis C	Inhibits viral RNA polymerases and end-capping of viral RNA	Myelosuppression, teratogenicity

J. Miscellaneous Antiviral Drugs
    1. Miscellaneous antiviral drugs are listed in Table 8–1.
    2. Table 8–1 provides the clinical uses, mechanisms of action, and toxicities for these drugs.

HIGHLY ACTIVE ANTIRETROVIRAL THERAPY (HAART)

- *Combination anti-HIV drug protocols commonly involve two nucleoside reverse transcriptase inhibitors plus a protease inhibitor.*
- *HAART slows the development of resistance and reverses the decline in CD4 cells that occurs during disease progression.*
- *Viral RNA load decreases (sometimes to undetectable levels) and the opportunistic infection rate is reduced by combination drug treatment.*
- *However, cessation of drug therapy in AIDS patients usually results in re-emergence of detectable viral RNA.*

III. Antiparasitic Drugs
    A. Antimalarial drugs are listed in Table 8–2.
    B. Drugs for specific protozoal infections are listed in Table 8–3.
    C. Anthelmintic drugs include drugs for nematode infections (Table 8–4) and drugs for trematode and cestode infections (Table 8–5).

GLUCOSE-6-PHOSPHATE DEHYDROGENASE DEFICIENCY

- *Patients with this common X-linked enzymopathy are susceptible to attacks of acute hemolysis if exposed to chemicals that cause oxidative stress.*
- *The disease is most prevalent in males of African, Asian, or Mediterranean descent.*

Table 8–2. Antimalarial drugs.

Drug	Mechanisms of Action	Clinical Uses	Toxicities
Chloroquine	Heme accumulation; resistance via efflux transporters	Prophylaxis and treatment in chloroquine-sensitive regions	Gastrointestinal distress, skin rash, and at high doses neuropathy, retinopathy, auditory dysfunction, and psychosis
Atovaquone + proguanil	Inhibit mitochondrial electron transport and folate metabolism	Chloroquine-resistant malaria	Rash, cough and gastrointestinal effects; avoid in pregnancy and in severe renal dysfunction
Mefloquine[1]	Chemically related to chloroquine, but mechanism unknown	Chloroquine-resistant malaria	Gastrointestinal, skin rash and headache; avoid if history of seizures
Primaquine	Forms redox compounds that cause cellular oxidation	*Plasmodium vivax* and *P ovale*	Gastrointestinal distress, pruritus, headache, methemoglobinemia; avoid in G6PD deficiency
Quinine	Blocks DNA replication and transcription to RNA	Chloroquine-resistant *Plasmodium falciparum*	Cinchonism, quinidinelike cardiotoxicity, and blackwater fever; avoid in pregnancy and in G6PD deficiency.

[1]Mefloquine is a drug of choice for prophylaxis in chloroquine-resistant regions; doxycycline and atovaquone-proguanil (Malarone) are also used and have activity in malaria caused by mefloquine-resistant falciparum malaria.

- Antimalarial drugs to be avoided in G6PD deficiency include chloroquine, primaquine, and quinine.
- Other drugs that are contraindicated in G6PD deficiency include α-methyldopa, chloramphenicol, dimercaprol, enalapril, hydralazine, nitrofurantoin, norfloxacin, primaquine, procainamide, probenecid, quinidine, and antibacterial sulfonamides.

HELMINTIC INFECTIONS

- Over one billion persons worldwide are estimated to be infected with intestinal nematodes and half that number suffer from tissue nematode infections.

Table 8–3. Drugs for specific protozoal infections.

Infection	Primary Drug s)	Comments
Amebiasis	Metronidazole	Diloxanide (or iodoquinol) can be used for noninvasive intestinal disease
Giardiasis	Metronidazole	"Backpacker's diarrhea" may not need drug treatment
Leishmaniasis	Stibogluconate	Metronidazole, pentamidine, and polyenes are back-up drugs
Pneumocystosis	TMP-SMX	Aerosolic pentamidine is also prophylactic, but the intravenous form is needed for treatment; atovaquone is also active
Trichomoniasis	Metronidazole	Treat both sexual partners
Toxoplasmosis	Pyrimethamine + sulfadiazine	Clindamycin is a back-up drug if sulfonamides are contraindicated
Trypanosomiasis	Melarsoprol Nifurtimox	African forms American forms

- In the United States pinworm infections are common, with hookworm and threadworm infection endemic in the southern states.
- Trematodes (flukes) are endemic in Southeast Asia and the Indian subcontinent.
- Cestode (tapeworm) infections occur in most world regions.

CLINICAL PROBLEMS

A young male patient who has no prior history of HSV infection develops painful pustular lesions on his genitalia and severe dysuria with a mucoid discharge characteristic of herpetic urethritis. Acyclovir is prescribed for his condition.

1. Which of the following statements about acyclovir and its use in this patient is accurate?

   A. Acyclovir must be administered intravenously in herpetic urethritis

   B. Dose-dependent bone marrow suppression is anticipated with the use of acyclovir

   C. Once-daily oral dosing with acyclovir is effective in genitourinary herpes infections

   D. Thymidine kinase–deficient strains of HSV are resistant to acyclovir

   E. To prevent crystalluria this patient should be administered mannitol parenterally

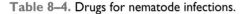

Table 8–4. Drugs for nematode infections.

Drug	Infections	Characteristics and Comments
Albendazole	Co-drug of choice for most common nematodes	Inhibits microtubule assembly in worms
Dimethylcarbamazine	Drug of choice for filariasis	Reactions to parasite proteins include fever, rashes, joint pain, and ocular dysfunction
Ivermectin	Drug of choice for threadworm	GABA receptor activation leads to paralysis and expulsion of worms
Mebendazole	Drug of choice for whipworm; co-drug of choice for hookworm, pin-worm, and round-worm	Inhibits microtubule synthesis in worms; avoid in pregnancy
Piperazine	Back-up drug for roundworm	GABA receptor activation leads to paralysis and expulsion of worms
Pyrantel pamoate	Co-drug of choice for hookworm and roundworm	Nicotinic receptor activation causes a depolarization paralysis of worms
Thiabendazole	Drug of choice for larva migrans	Toxicity includes gastrointestinal dis-tress, cholestasis, leukopenia, CNS effects, and reactions to dying parasites

2. Influenza vaccines are contraindicated in patients with egg allergy. In such cases pro-phylaxis against influenza types A and B can be provided by which of the following?

    A. Amantadine

    B. Foscarnet

    C. Oseltamivir

    D. Ribavirin

    E. Valacyclovir

A 37-year-old female patient who has been treated for Hodgkin's disease is cellularly immun-odeficient. She develops symptoms of headache, confusion, nausea, and vomiting. Spinal fluid findings include increased pressure, pleocytosis, increased protein, decreased glucose, and budding encapsulated fungal cells. A preliminary diagnosis of fungal meningitis is made and CSF analysis demonstrates polysaccharide antigen of Cryptococcus neoformans.

Table 8–5. Drugs for trematode and cestode infections.

Drug	Infections	Characteristics and Comments
Bithionol	Drug of choice for sheep liver fluke	Causes tinnitus, headache, phototoxicity, gastrointestinal distress, and leukopenia
Metrifonate	Bilharziasis	Inhibits acetylcholinesterase of parasites
Praziquantel	Drug of choice for most flukes and co-drug of choice for most tapeworms	Increases Ca^{2+} influx causing parasite contraction then relaxation; causes headache, dizziness, malaise, and gastrointestinal distress
Albendazole	Drug of choice for cystercercosis and hydatid disease	See Table 8–4
Niclosamide	Co-drug of choice for most tapeworms	Uncouples oxidative phosphorylation; causes headache, gastrointestinal distress, rashes, and fever

3. Which of the following statements about the management of this patient is accurate?

   A. Amphotericin B (intrathecal) must be administered in all cases of cryptococcal meningitis

   B. The antifungal drug treatment of choice is monotherapy with flucytosine at maximally tolerated doses

   C. In patients with mild disease (spinal fluid antigen titer < 1:128) oral fluconazole for 12 weeks is an effective treatment regimen

   D. Ketoconazole has synergistic effects with amphotericin B in the treatment of fungal meningitis due to *Cryptococcus neoformans*

   E. Terbinafine is highly effective in fungal meningitis, as it readily enters the CSF

4. If amphotericin B is used in the treatment of this patient, its potential nephrotoxic effects include azotemia, hypokalemia, hyposthenuria, nephrolithiasis, acute tubular necrosis, and renal failure. Nephrotoxicity of amphotericin B can be reduced by the use of which of the following?

   A. Antihistamines

   B. Hydrocortisone

   C. Ibuprofen

   D. Liposomal formulations

   E. Meperidine

A 30-year-old male patient with AIDS has a $CD4^+$ of 200/μL and a viral RNA load of 70,000 copies/mL. His highly active antiretroviral therapy (HAART) includes zidovudine, didanosine, and ritonavir. He has experienced several episodes of oral candidiasis that have been managed by treatment with ketoconazole. Oral trimethoprim-sulfamethoxazole (TMP-SMX) has been prescribed recently for prophylaxis against Pneumocystis carinii pneumonia. He is also taking dronabinol to improve appetite and decrease nausea.

5. In terms of drug toxicities he is likely to be experiencing, which of the following pairs of drug: adverse effect is accurate?

   A. Didanosine: hemolysis in G6PD deficiency

   B. Dronabinol: bone marrow suppression

   C. Ritonavir: inhibition of hepatic drug-metabolizing enzymes

   D. TMP-SMX: pancreatitis

   E. Zidovudine: gynecomastia

6. If this AIDS patient could not tolerate TMP-SMX because he was allergic to sulfon-amides, which of the following drugs would provide effective prophylaxis against *Pneumocystis carinii* pneumonia?

   A. Ampicillin

   B. Clarithromycin

   C. Nystatin

   D. Pentamidine

   E. Rifabutin

7. Which of the following is the optimal drug treatment of hepatic amebiasis?

   A. Diloxanide furoate

   B. Metronidazole

   C. Metronidazole plus a luminal amebicide

   D. Pyrantel pamoate

   E. Tetracycline

A person is advised to take 100 mg of doxycycline daily while visiting a foreign country.

8. This regimen will be an effective prophylaxis against which of the following?

   A. Ascariasis (roundworm infection)

   B. Malaria

   C. Tapeworm infections

   D. Sexually transmitted diseases

   E. Trypanosomiasis (sleeping sickness)

ANSWERS

1. The answer is D. Oral acyclovir is effective in genitourinary herpes infections, but the drug must be taken five times daily. Acyclovir is not hematotoxic and crystalluria is unlikely, especially after oral administration, if the patient maintains adequate hydration. HSV strains resistant to acyclovir commonly lack thymidine kinase, a viral enzyme that catalyzes the initial phosphorylation of the drug.

2. The answer is C. Taken orally (once daily) oseltamivir, a neuraminidase inhibitor, is effective in preventing influenza types A and B. Zanamivir, another neuraminidase inhibitor, is also effective. Amantadine is used for prophylaxis against and treatment of influenza A, but the drug is not effective against influenza B. Foscarnet and valacyclovir are used for herpetic infections. The clinical uses of ribavirin include management of infections due to respiratory syncytial virus (RSV) and adjunctive use with interferon-alfa in hepatitis C.

3. The answer is C. Oral fluconazole is used for prophylaxis and suppression in cryptococcal meningitis and is also effective for short-term treatment in mild cases. Intrathecal administration of amphotericin B is not mandatory in cryptococcal meningitis. Flucytosine has synergistic effects with amphotericin B, but would not be used as monotherapy due to rapid emergence of resistance. Ketoconazole has no activity against *Cryptococcus neoformans.* The antifungal activity of terbinafine is restricted to dermatophytes.

4. The answer is D. Antihistamines, glucocorticoids, nonsteroidal anti-inflammatory drugs (NSAIDs), and meperidine are commonly used to decrease the infusion-related toxicities of amphotericin B, which include headache, chills, fever, rigors, hypotension, and nausea and vomiting. None of these drugs affords protection against dose-limiting nephrotoxicity, but the incidence and severity of renal toxicity is reduced by the use of liposomal formulations of amphotericin B.

5. The answer is C. Ritonavir causes many drug interactions due to its inhibitory effects on hepatic drug-metabolizing enzymes. In the AIDS patient sulfonamides may cause hemolysis in G6PD deficiency. The hematotoxicity of zidovudine may require blood transfusions. Gynecomastia is an adverse effect of ketoconazole via its inhibition of gonadal hormone synthesis. The anti-HIV drug most likely to cause pancreatitis is didanosine.

6. The answer is D. Pentamidine or primaquine plus clindamycin is effective both in prophylaxis and treatment of infections caused by *Pneumocystis carinii.*

7. The answer is C. Metronidazole is the drug of choice for treatment of amebiasis and other extraintestinal infections due to *Entamoeba histolytica.* It is used together with a luminal amebicide such as diloxanide. Pyrantel pamoate is used for hookworm and roundworm infections.

8. The answer is B. Whereas mefloquine (weekly) is commonly used for prophylaxis against malaria in regions in which chloroquine resistance is endemic, doxycycline (daily) is also effective. Tetracyclines are not reliably prophylactic against sexually transmitted diseases and they do not protect against worm infections or sleeping sickness.

CHAPTER 9
ANTICANCER DRUGS AND IMMUNO-PHARMACOLOGY

I. Cancer Chemotherapy

A. Concepts

1. **Cell cycle kinetics:** Cell cycle–specific (CCS) drugs act on tumor cells during the mitotic cycle and are usually phase specific (Figure 9–1). Most anticancer drugs are cell cycle–nonspecific (CCNS), killing tumor cells in both resting and cycling phases.

2. **Log kill:** Antitumor drug treatment kills a fixed **proportion** of a cancer cell population rather than a constant number of cells. A 3-log-kill dose of a drug reduces cancer cell numbers by three orders of magnitude.

3. **Resistance:** Established mechanisms of tumor cell resistance to anticancer drugs are shown in Table 9–1.

4. **Toxicities:** Drug-specific toxicities are given in Table 9–2.

TOXICITY OF ANTICANCER DRUGS

CLINICAL CORRELATION

- *Normal cells with a high growth fraction (bone marrow, gastrointestinal mucosa, ovaries, and hair follicles) are highly susceptible to the cytotoxic actions of anticancer drugs.*

- *Bone marrow suppression is common with both alkylating agents and antimetabolites; it is often the dose-limiting toxicity.*

- *Drug dosage is usually titrated to avoid excessive neutropenia (granulocytes < 500/dL) or thrombocytopenia (platelets < 20,000/dL).*

- *The use of colony-stimulating factors decreases the infection rate and the need for antibiotics.*

B. Alkylating Agents

1. **Mechanisms of action:** The **alkylating agents** are CCNS drugs.
   a. They interact covalently with DNA bases, especially at the N-7 position of guanine.
   b. Nucleic acid functions are disrupted due to cross-linking, abnormal base pairing, and DNA strand breakage.

2. **Cisplatin** and **carboplatin** form cytotoxic free radicals; they are used in regimens for cancers of the bladder, lung, ovary, and testes.

3. **Cyclophosphamide** is activated via hepatic cytochrome P-450 (CYP450) enzymes, but forms acrolein, causing bladder toxicity; it is used in regimens for breast and ovarian cancers and non-Hodgkin's lymphoma.

4. **Nitrosureas** (**carmustine** and **lomustine**) are highly lipid soluble and penetrate into the CNS; they are used adjunctively in brain tumors.

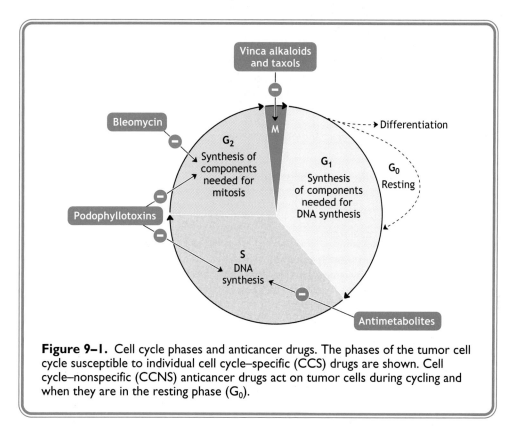

Figure 9–1. Cell cycle phases and anticancer drugs. The phases of the tumor cell cycle susceptible to individual cell cycle–specific (CCS) drugs are shown. Cell cycle–nonspecific (CCNS) anticancer drugs act on tumor cells during cycling and when they are in the resting phase (G_0).

Table 9–1. Resistance to anticancer drugs.

Mechanisms of Resistance	Anticancer Drugs Affected
Increased DNA repair	Alkylating agents
Formation of trapping agents	Alkylating agents
Changes in target enzymes or receptors	Etoposide, gonadal hormones, methotrexate, vincristine, vinblastine
Decreased activation of prodrugs	6-Mercaptopurine, 5-fluorouracil
Formation of drug-inactivating enzymes	Purine and pyrimidine antimetabolites
Decreased drug accumulation via increase in P-glycoprotein transporters	Alkylating agents, dactinomycin, methotrexate

Table 9–2. Anticancer drug-specific toxicities.

Drug	Specific Toxicities
Bleomycin[1]	Pulmonary fibrosis, fevers, skin hardening and blisters, anaphylaxis
Cisplatin[1]	Nephrotoxicity, acoustic and peripheral neuropathy
Cyclophosphamide	Hemorrhagic cystitis—mesna is protective (traps acrolein); ifosfamide is similar to cyclophosphamide
Doxorubicin and daunorubicin	Cardiomyopathy (eg, delayed heart failure)—dexrazoxane is protective (decreases free radical formation); liposomal forms are less cardiotoxic
Methotrexate (MTX)	Myelosuppression (use "leucovorin rescue") and mucositis; crystalluria; toxicity is enhanced by drugs that displace MTX from plasma proteins (eg, salicylates, sulfonamides)
Vincristine[1]	Peripheral neuropathy (autonomic, motor, and sensory); vinblastine is less neurotoxic; paclitaxel also causes sensory neuropathy

[1]Bone marrow-sparing drugs.

  5. Procarbazine forms free radicals; it is used in Hodgkin's lymphoma, but may cause leukemia.
C. **Antimetabolites**
  1. **Mechanisms of action:** Antimetabolites are CCS drugs.
    a. They are structurally similar to endogenous compounds.
    b. Anticancer and immunosuppressive actions result from interference with the metabolic functions of folic acid, purines, and pyrimidines.
  2. **Methotrexate (MTX)** is an analog of folic acid that inhibits dihydrofolate reductase and other enzymes in folic acid metabolism.
    a. It is used (orally and intravenously) in acute leukemias, breast cancers, and non-Hodgkin's and T-cell lymphomas.
    b. **Folinic acid (leucovorin)** is used to reverse MTX toxicities and full hydration is needed to prevent crystalluria.
  3. **Mercaptopurine (6-MP)** inhibits purine metabolism following its activation by hypoxanthine guanine phosphoribosyl transferase (HGPRT).
    a. Resistant cells may lack HGPRT.
    b. 6-MP is used mainly in regimens for acute leukemias.
  4. **Cytarabine (Ara-C)** is activated by tumor cell kinases to form a nucleotide that inhibits pyrimidine metabolism.
    a. Resistant cells may lack such kinases.
    b. Ara-C is used mainly in regimens for acute leukemias.

5. Fluorouracil (5-FU) is activated to a metabolite that inhibits thymidylate synthase causing "thymine-less death" of tumor cells.
    a. Changes in this enzyme may result in resistance.
    b. 5-FU is widely used, mainly for the treatment of solid tumors.

MULTIDRUG RESISTANCE

CLINICAL
CORRELATION

- *Resistance to multiple anticancer drugs may occur from increased expression of the MDRI gene for cell surface glycoproteins (P-glycoproteins) involved in drug efflux.*
- *Such drug transporters (not limited to cancer cells) use ATP to drive drug molecules out of a cell against a concentration gradient.*
- *Verapamil (a calcium channel antagonist) inhibits these drug transporters.*

D. Plant Alkaloids (CCS Drugs)
    1. Etoposide and **teniposide** act in late S and early G_2 phases, inhibiting topoisomerases.
        a. They are used in regimens for lung (small cell), prostate, and testicular cancers.
        b. These agents cause myelosuppression.
    2. Paclitaxel and **docetaxel** act in the M phase to block mitotic spindle disassembly.
        a. They are used in advanced breast and ovarian cancers.
        b. Significant myelosuppression occurs, but peripheral neuropathy is distinctive.
    3. Vinblastine and **vincristine** act in the M phase to block mitotic spindle assembly.
        a. They are widely used in combination regimens for acute leukemias, Hodgkin's and other lymphomas, Kaposi's sarcoma, neuroblastoma, and testicular cancer.
        b. Vincristine is neurotoxic.
        c. Vinblastine suppresses bone marrow.

E. Antibiotics
    1. Bleomycin is a glycopeptide mixture (CCS) that alters nucleic acid functions via free radical formation.
        a. It is used in regimens for Hodgkin's and other lymphomas and squamous cell and testicular cancers.
        b. Pulmonary toxicity, skin thickening, and hypersensitivity reactions are distinctive.
    2. Doxorubicin and **daunorubicin** are anthracyclines (CCNS) that intercalate with DNA, inhibit topisomerases, and form free radicals.
        a. Doxorubicin is widely used in breast, endometrial, lung, and ovarian cancers and in Hodgkin's lymphoma.
        b. Daunorubicin is used in leukemias.
        c. Myelosuppression is marked, but cardiotoxicity is dose limiting.
    3. Other antibiotics include **dactinomycin** and **mitomycin.**
        a. Dactinomycin (CCNS) inhibits DNA-dependent RNA synthesis and is used in melanoma and Wilms' tumors.
        b. Mitomycin (CCNS) is biotransformed to an alkylating agent and is used for hypoxic tumors.
        c. Both of these agents cause bone marrow suppression.

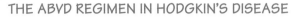

THE ABVD REGIMEN IN HODGKIN'S DISEASE

- *Chemotherapy in cancer commonly involves the use of drug combinations to enhance antitumor actions and to prevent development of resistance.*
- *The **ABVD regimen** includes **doxorubicin (Adriamycin), bleomycin, vinblastine,** and **dacarbazine** (an alkylating agent).*
- *This drug regimen, used in cycles with total nodal radiotherapy, has achieved up to 80% remission in stages III and IV of Hodgkin's disease.*
- *Toxicities, which can be severe, include alopecia, gastrointestinal distress, neutropenia, thrombocytopenia, and possible sterility.*
- *In addition, patients on the ABVD regimen may suffer the pulmonary toxicity of bleomycin and a delayed cardiomyopathy caused by doxorubicin.*

    F. **Hormones**
       1. **Glucocorticoids** include **prednisone,** which is used in combination regimens for Hodgkin's lymphoma and leukemias.
       2. **Gonadal hormones** include the palliative use (rare) of androgens in estrogen-dependent cancers in women and the use of estrogens in prostate cancer.
       3. **Gonadal hormone antagonists** include estrogen receptor blockers (**tamoxifen** and **toremifene**) and the androgen receptor blocker **flutamide.** They are used for tumors responsive to gonadal hormones.
       4. **Gonadotropin-releasing hormone analogs** include **leuprolide** and **naferelin,** which decrease follicle-stimulating hormone (FSH) and luteinizing hormone (LH) if used in constant doses.
       5. **Aromatase inhibitors** include **anastrozole,** which inhibits formation of estrogens from androstenedione and is used in advanced breast cancer.
    G. **Miscellaneous Anticancer Agents**
       1. **Asparaginase** depletes serum asparagine and is used in auxotrophic T-cell leukemias and lymphomas. It causes bleeding, hypersensitivity reactions, and pancreatitis.
       2. **Interferons** include interferon-alfa, which is used in early-stage chronic myelogenous leukemia, hairy cell cancers, and T-cell lymphomas. Interferons cause myelosuppression and neurotoxicity.
       3. **Monoclonal antibodies.**
          a. **Gemtuzumab** interacts with the CD33 antigen and is used in CD33$^+$ myeloid leukemias; severe myelosuppression is the major toxicity.
          b. **Rituximab** interacts with a surface protein of non-Hodgkin's lymphoma cells; toxicities include myelosuppression and hypersensitivity reactions.
          c. **Trastuzumab** is used for breast tumors that overexpress the HER2 protein; toxicity includes cardiac dysfunction.
          d. **Alemtuzumab,** which targets the CD52 antigen, is used for treatment of B-cell chronic lymphocytic leukemia (CLL).
       4. **Imatinib** is a protein designed to inhibit the abnormal tyrosine kinase created by the Philadelphia chromosome abnormality in chronic myelogenous leukemia (CML); toxicity includes diarrhea, myalgia, and fluid retention.
  II. **Immunopharmacology**
    A. **Concepts**
       1. Most immunosuppressant drugs interfere with the proliferation of B-lymphoid cells (mediators of humoral immunity and antibody formation) and T-lymphoid cells (mediators of cellular immunity) (Figure 9–2).

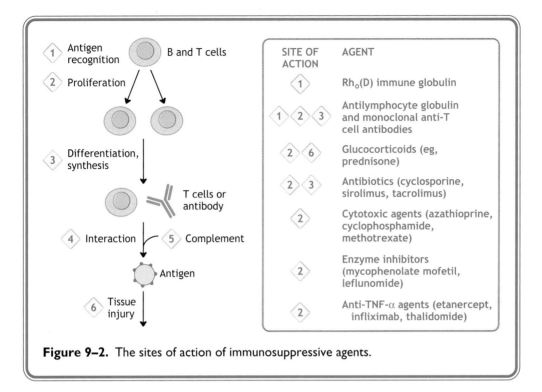

Figure 9–2. The sites of action of immunosuppressive agents.

    2. Antibodies also inhibit antigen recognition, and like some antibiotics (eg, cyclosporine), have inhibitory effects on lymphoid cell differentiation.

    3. Glucocorticoids inhibit lymphocyte proliferation, but also protect against late-developing biochemical events that result in tissue injury.

B. Cyclosporine & Related Immunosuppressive Drugs

    1. Mechanisms of action: Cyclosporine binds to cyclophilin and the complex inhibits calcineurin, a cytoplasmic phosphatase that activates T-cell transcription factors, leading to decreases in cytokines including interleukin-2 and interferon-alfa. **Tacrolimus** has a similar action but binds to FK-binding protein (FK-BP) to inhibit calcineurin. **Sirolimus** also binds to FK-BP but inhibits mTor (a protein kinase) leading to decreased synthesis of interleukins and γ-globulins.

    2. Clinical uses: Cyclosporine, the prototype, has been the major immunosuppressant drug in organ and tissue transplantation; tacrolimus and sirolimus appear to have equivalent efficacy in most situations.

    3. Toxicities: Cyclosporine and tacrolimus cause nephrotoxicity, peripheral neuropathy, and hypertension; sirolimus causes hyperlipidemia and hematotoxicity.

C. Other Immunosuppressive Drugs

    1. Glucocorticoids inhibit the formation of prostaglandins and leukotrienes and decrease platelet-activating factor and interleukins (eg, interleukin-2).

        a. Pharmacologic doses are used for immunosuppressive and anti-inflammatory effects.

        b. Glucocorticoids are used in a wide range of autoimmune diseases and adjunctively in transplantation.

2. **Mycophenolate mofetil** suppresses B and T lymphocyte proliferation via inhibition of inosine monophosphate dehydrogenase, preventing the formation of purines.
   a. It is used as a primary drug in transplantation.
   b. It decreases cyclosporine dose requirement (and nephrotoxicity) if used in combination.
3. **Azathioprine** forms mercaptopurine, which, after bioactivation, inhibits purine synthesis.
   a. It is used mainly in autoimmune diseases.
   b. Myelosuppression is the main toxicity.
4. **Etanercept** is a recombinant form of the tumor necrosis factor (TNF) receptor that binds TNF and prevents its actions.
   a. It is used in rheumatoid arthritis.
   b. Toxicity includes hypersensitivity reactions and infections.
5. **Leflunomide** decreases ribonucleotide synthesis in lymphocytes via inhibition of dihydroorotic acid dehydrogenase.
   a. It is used in rheumatoid arthritis.
   b. Toxicities include alopecia, rash, and hepatotoxicity.
6. **Thalidomide** suppresses the activity of TNF.
   a. It is used in systemic lupus erythematosus and for aphthous ulcers and the wasting syndrome in AIDS patients.
   b. Thalidomide is strongly teratogenic.

ALLERGIC RHINITIS

CLINICAL
CORRELATION

- *Drugs used for this immunoglobulin E (IgE)-mediated condition can inhibit mediator release from mast cells, interfere with mediator actions on target cells, or protect target tissues against inflammatory and vascular responses.*
- *Agents commonly used include the antihistamines, sympathomimetics (decongestants and bronchodilators), and glucocorticoids.*
- *Mast cell stabilizers and inhaled muscarinic receptor blockers also have value in some patients.*
- *Immunotherapy (long-term allergen injection) is effective in patients who respond poorly to drugs and whose allergens are unavoidable.*

  D. Antibodies
1. **Antilymphocytic globulin (ALG)** is an equine antibody that blocks cellular immunity and is used to suppress organ graft rejection; drug reactions include serum sickness and vasculitis.
2. **$Rh_o(D)$ immune globulin (Rh_oGAM)**, which contains antibodies against red cell $Rh_o(D)$ antigens, is used in $Rh_o(D)$-negative pregnant women at the birth of an $Rh_o(D)$-positive child to prevent hemolytic disease of the newborn in subsequent pregnancies.
3. Several **monoclonal antibodies (MAbs)** are used in cancer chemotherapy.
   a. **Abciximab,** a MAb that binds to the glycoprotein IIIb/IIa receptor, is used as an antiplatelet agent.
   b. **Daclizumab,** a blocker of interleukin-2 receptors, has adjunctive use in renal transplantation; basiliximab is similar.
   c. In Crohn's disease and rheumatoid arthritis **infliximab** neutralizes tumor necrosis factor.

Table 9–3. Recombinant cytokines and clinical uses.

Agent	Clinical Uses
Aldesleukin (interleukin-2)	Renal cell carcinoma, metastatic melanoma
Erythropoietin	Anemias (especially in renal failure)
Filgrastim (granulocyte colony-stimulating factor)	Recovery of bone marrow
Interferon-alpha	Hepatitis B and C, Kaposi's sarcoma, leukemias, malignant melanoma
Interferon-beta	Multiple sclerosis
Interferon-gamma	Chronic granulomatous disease
Oprelvekin (interleukin-11)	Thrombocytopenia
Sargramostim (granulocyte-macrophage colony stimulating factor	Recovery of bone marrow
Thrombopoietin	Thrombocytopenia

       d. Palivizumab interacts with a protein component of respiratory syncytial virus (RSV), and is used for its prophylaxis and treatment

E. Immunomodulators
  1. Many cytokines and lymphokines modulate immune and/or inflammatory responses, including interferons, interleukins, and colony-stimulating factors.
  2. Through recombinant DNA technology a number of these natural compounds are available for use as pharmacologic agents (Table 9–3).

F. Drug Allergy
  1. Immunologic reactions to drugs can be classified into four types: I–IV.
  2. These are summarized in Table 9–4.

CLINICAL PROBLEMS

Having undergone surgery for breast cancer, a 46-year-old female patient is to receive a course of chemotherapy with a regimen that includes cyclophosphamide, methotrexate, fluorouracil, and tamoxifen.

1. Which of the following compounds offers protection for this patient against hemorrhagic cystitis, a common toxicity of cyclophosphamide?

Table 9–4. Allergic reactions to drugs.

Type	Reaction and Causative Drugs
Type I (immediate); IgE-mediated release of inflammatory mediators	Anaphylaxis, angioedema, urticaria; caused by many drugs, especially penicillins and sulfonamides
Type II (autoimmune); IgG or IgM complement-dependent cell lysis	Agranulocytosis (clozapine), drug-induced lupus (procainamide), hemolytic anemia (methyldopa), thrombocytopenic purpura (quinidine)
Type III; multi system, complement-fixing IgG or IgM antibodies	Serum sickness and vasculitis (penicillins, sulfonamides, phenytoin, iodide); Stevens–Johnson syndrome (sulfonamides, lamotrigine)
Type IV; cell-mediated skin reactions	Contact dermatitis (neomycin)

    A. Aldesleukin

    B. Dexrazoxane

    C. Folinic acid

    D. Mesna

    E. Vitamin B_6

2. If the tumor cells responsible for breast cancer in this patient have a form of thymidylate synthase that is drug resistant, which component(s) of the proposed regimen is unlikely to have anticancer activity?

    A. Cyclophosphamide

    B. Fluorouracil

    C. Methotrexate

    D. Tamoxifen

    E. All of the above

3. Which of the following anticancer drugs is cell cycle–specific (CCS) and causes hypersensitivity reactions, skin changes, and pulmonary fibrosis?

    A. Bleomycin

    B. Busulfan

    C. Cisplatin

    D. Methotrexate

    E. Vincristine

A 35-year-old male patient undergoing chemotherapy for testicular cancer has muscle weakness manifest by difficulty in standing up from a sitting position. He also has constipation.

4. If his problems are drug related which of the following anticancer drugs is most likely to be responsible?

   A. Bleomycin

   B. Flutamide

   C. Leuprolide

   D. Paclitaxel

   E. Vincristine

A patient with rheumatoid arthritis develops tuberculosis soon after he starts using a new drug that specifically acts by interfering with tumor necrosis factor.

5. This patient is being treated with which of the following?

   A. Aldesleukin

   B. Infliximab

   C. Leflunomide

   D. Mycophenolate mofetil

   E. Trastuzumab

Prior to bone marrow transplantation a patient is treated with antilymphocytic globulin (ALG). He develops erythematous skin eruptions, fever, lymphadenopathy, and arthralgia, that appear to be due to a drug reaction.

6. Which of the following statements about this case is accurate?

   A. Corticosteroids will intensify these symptoms

   B. Epinephrine should be administered immediately

   C. Antilymphocytic globulin frequently causes type II autoimmune reactions

   D. The patient is suffering from serum sickness

   E. This is a type IV drug allergy

7. Which of the following agents is effective in preventing rejection in organ transplantation and is much less toxic than immunosuppressive antibiotics or glucocorticoids?

   A. Azathioprine

   B. Cyclophosphamide

   C. Mycophenolate mofetil

   D. Rituximab

   E. Tacrolimus

Drug-induced lupus differs from systemic lupus erythematosus (SLE) by its lack of gender bias, by its infrequent presentation of severe renal and neurologic symptoms, and by the reversal of symptoms on drug withdrawal.

8. Drug-induced lupus has been definitely associated with the use of which of the following?

   A. Hydralazine

   B. Methyldopa

C. Procainamide

D. Quinidine

E. All of the above

ANSWERS

1. The answer is D. Mesna (mercaptoethanesulfonate) forms a complex with acrolein, the metabolite of cyclophosphamide that causes bladder toxicity. Aldesleukin is a recombinant form of interleukin-2; dexrazoxane blocks the formation of free radicals that are responsible for the cardiotoxicity of doxorubicin; folinic acid is used to reverse methotrexate toxicity; vitamin B_6 protects against the peripheral neurotoxicity of isoniazid.

2. The answer is B. Fluorouracil (5-FU) is biotransformed to 5-fluorodeoxyuridine monophosphate (5-FdUMP), which inhibits thymidylate synthase and causes a "thymine-less death" of tumor cells. One mechanism of resistance to 5-FU involves changes in the gene that encodes thymidylate synthase, leading either to an increase in the synthesis of the enzyme or a decrease in its sensitivity to inhibition by 5-FdUMP.

3. The answer is A. Pulmonary dysfunction occurs with very few anticancer drugs. Bleomycin is the anticancer drug most commonly associated with causing pulmonary fibrosis. Dermatotoxicity and pulmonary dysfunction are also known adverse effects of busulfan. However, busulfan is cell cycle–nonspecific (CCNS) and compared with bleomycin is used very infrequently. None of the other drugs listed, all of which are cell cycle–specific (CCS), causes pulmonary dysfunction.

4. The answer is E. Vinca alkaloids are well-accepted components of curative chemotherapy regimens in testicular cancer. Vincristine causes autonomic and motor neuropathy with symptoms of constipation and muscle weakness. Cisplatin (not listed), also a component of regimens used for testicular cancer, causes sensory neuropathy including deafness. Paclitaxel causes mainly sensory neuropathy and is used in the treatment of advanced breast and ovarian cancer.

5. The answer is B. Infliximab and etanercept (not listed) both interfere with the activity of tumor necrosis factor (TNF). Their use in rheumatoid arthritis (RA) is associated with an increased infection rate. Leflunomide is also used in RA, but inhibits ribonucleotide synthesis and has no effects on TNF.

6. The answer is D. The symptoms are those of serum sickness, a type III drug reaction associated with exposure to many drugs including foreign antibodies such as antilymphocytic globulin (ALG). The symptoms subside slowly when the offending agent is withdrawn and corticosteroids are usually ameliorative. Epinephrine is used for type I allergic reactions (eg, anaphylaxis). Types II and IV drug reactions are not associated with the clinical use of ALG.

7. The answer is C. Mycophenolate mofetil is an effective immunosuppressant in organ transplantation with adverse effects limited to gastrointestinal distress. Although an-

timetabolites (eg, azathioprine) and cytotoxic drugs (eg, cyclophosphamide) are also used to prevent rejection, they cause severe hematotoxicity. The toxic effects of tacrolimus, like those of cyclosporine, include renal dysfunction and peripheral neuropathy.

8. The answer is E. Drug-induced lupus (a type II reaction) also differs from SLE in that hypocomplementemia and antibodies to native DNA are absent.

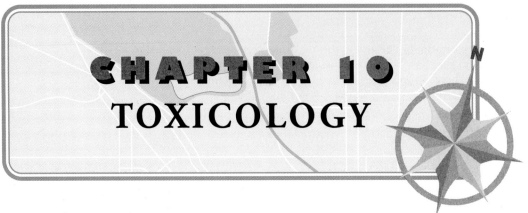

CHAPTER 10
TOXICOLOGY

I. Introduction

A. Concepts

1. **Toxicology** is the branch of pharmacology that studies the **adverse effects of chemicals on biological systems.**
2. **Clinical toxicology** concerns the adverse effects of pharmacologic agents and includes toxicity testing of new drugs.
3. Toxicology also includes the identification and management of **environmental and occupational chemical hazards,** such as air pollutants, agricultural chemicals, waste products of the chemical industry, and heavy metals.

B. Toxicity Testing of New Drugs

1. The Food and Drug Administration (FDA) requires acute and chronic toxicity studies in animals of new drugs that are intended for chronic systemic use in humans (preclinical animal studies).
2. Toxicity testing (in two animal species) usually involves assessments of drug effects on blood, cardiovascular, hepatic, pulmonary, and renal functions.
3. Gross and histopathologic examinations of tissues are required, as are tests of reproductive effects and potential carcinogenicity.

II. Environmental Chemicals

A. Air Pollutants

1. Industrial air pollutants, including carbon monoxide (50%), oxides of nitrogen and sulfur (25%), hydrocarbons (13%), and particulate matter (12%), are contributory factors in cardiopulmonary disease.
2. **Carbon monoxide (CO)** is an odorless, colorless gas that competes with oxygen for binding to hemoglobin and causes tissue hypoxia.
   a. Symptoms of exposure range from headache and malaise to mental confusion, tachycardia, syncope, acidosis, coma, and seizures.
   b. Most CO poisoning occurs from automobile exhausts and use of space heaters.
   c. Management involves removal from the source and use of pure oxygen; hyperbaric oxygen may be used in severe poisoning.
3. **Sulfur dioxide** (from fossil fuel combustion) is a conjunctival and bronchial irritant; **nitrogen dioxide** (formed from fires and farm silage) is a mucous membrane irritant and may cause pulmonary edema.
4. **Hydrocarbons** are commonly used as industrial solvents (eg, benzene, carbon tetrachloride, tetrachloroethylene, and toluene).

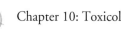

a. Short-term exposure causes central nervous system (CNS) depression.

b. Long-term exposure causes hematotoxicity (eg, benzene), nephrotoxicity, and hepatotoxicity.

c. The chlorinated hydrocarbons are also environmental pollutants (eg, DDT).

CYANIDE IN SMOKE

CLINICAL CORRELATION

- *Cyanide contributes to morbidity and mortality in smoke inhalation from fires in enclosed spaces.*
- *Many compounds produce cyanide gas when combusted, including household plastics and polyurethane.*
- *If cyanide toxicity is suspected, airway management with 100% oxygen and antidotal therapy with sodium nitrite should be initiated immediately.*
- *Bicarbonate for acidosis and anticonvulsants may also be used in management.*
- *Sodium nitrite converts hemoglobin to methemoglobin, which has a high affinity for cyanide, forming cyanomethemoglobin and thus preventing the binding of cyanide to cytochrome oxidase.*

B. Environmental Pollutants

1. **Dioxins: Polychlorinated dioxins** are by-products of the chemical industry that are resistant to environmental degradation.

   a. In animal studies dioxins cause multiple organ system toxicities and are both carcinogenic and teratogenic.

   b. Dioxins cause dermatotoxicity in humans and long-term exposure (eg, from groundwater) may be carcinogenic.

2. **Polychlorinated biphenyls (PCBs):** Formerly used in electrical equipment, the PCBs are resistant to degradation and accumulate in the food chain.

   a. Dermatotoxicity occurred in chemical workers exposed to PCBs.

   b. Changes in hepatic function and lipid metabolism are suspected.

III. Agricultural Chemicals

A. Insecticides

1. **Cholinesterase inhibitors: Carbamates** (eg, carbaryl) and **organophosphates** (eg, malathion) are widely used agricultural insecticides. Signs and symptoms of poisoning (see "DUMBBELSS" mnemonic in Table 10–3) are managed with atropine and the enzyme-reactivating agent pralidoxime (2-PAM). The same antidotal management would be applied in the case of exposure to nerve gases (eg, sarin) that inactivate acetylcholinesterase.

2. **Botanicals: Pyrethrums** cause neurotoxicity; **nicotine** activates N receptors at multiple sites; **rotenones** are gastrointestinal and skin irritants.

3. **Chlorinated hydrocarbons: Dichlorodiphenyltrichloroethane (DDT)** and related insecticides are resistant to environmental degradation and accumulate in the food chain.

   a. They are rarely used in North America.

   b. DDT is embryotoxic and carcinogenic in animals.

   c. Neurotoxicity occurs with acute exposure in humans.

B. Herbicides

1. **Paraquat:** This widely used agent causes acute gastrointestinal toxicity on ingestion (3–5 mL) and a delayed pulmonary fibrosis. There is no specific antidote.

2. **Phenoxyacetic acids:** Exposure to high doses from aerial spraying causes hypotonia and coma; long-term exposure may increase the risk of cancer.

Table 10–1. Heavy metal toxicities.

Metal	Sources	Signs and Symptoms
Arsenic	Insecticides, pesticides, wood preservatives, fossil fuels	*Acute:* gastrointestinal distress, "garlic" breath, "ricewater" stools *Chronic:* alopecia, anemia, carcinogenic
Iron	Medicinals, prenatal supplements	*Acute:* (mainly children): severe gastrointestinal distress, necrotizing gastroenteritis with hematemesis, bloody diarrhea, shock and coma
Lead	Paint chips (pica), tap water, herbals, glazed kitchenware	*Acute:* nausea and vomiting, malaise, tremor, tinnitus, paresthesias, encephalopathy *Chronic:* anemia, neuropathy ("wrist drop"), nephropathy, mental retardation, infertility
Mercury	Elemental in instruments; salts in amalgams, batteries, dyes, electroplating, photography	*Acute:* (vapor inhalation): chest pain, dyspnea, pneumonitis *Acute* (salts): gastrointestinal distress, bleeding, shock, renal failure

IV. Heavy Metals

    A. The **toxicities of heavy metals** differ, but their effects mainly result from their interactions with sulfhydryl groups on proteins (Table 10–1).

    B. **Chelating agents** interact with heavy metals and the complexes formed are readily eliminated (Table 10–2).

LEAD POISONING

CLINICAL CORRELATION

- *Ingestion of lead-based paint fragments (pica) in small children causes anemia, gastrointestinal irritation, growth retardation, neurocognitive deficits, and possibly encephalopathy.*
- *Lead toxicity via the oral route most commonly occurs in children living in homes constructed before 1950.*
- *A tentative diagnosis of lead poisoning may be confirmed by blood analysis of levels of lead > 20 μg/dL.*
- *Management involves removal from the source (if possible) and the oral use of succimer, a chelating agent.*

V. Management of Poisoning

    A. **Maintenance of Vital Functions**

        1. Maintenance of vital functions involves **ABCD: A**irway (open and protected), **B**reathing (effective ventilation), **C**irculation (circulatory support and correct arrhythmias), and **D**extrose.

        2. In suspected **alcoholism,** treat with **thiamine;** in suspected **opioid overdose,** treat with **naloxone.**

Table 10–2. Chelating agents.

Chelator	Clinical Uses	Toxicities
Deferoxamine	Iron poisoning	Hypotension if rapid intravenous administration; pulmonary and neurotoxicity if long-term treatment
Dimercaprol	Arsenic, lead, and mercury poisoning	Cardiovascular stimulation, gastrointestinal distress, and thrombocytopenia
EDTA[1]	Lead poisoning	Potentially nephrotoxic
Penicillamine	Copper poisoning or Wilson's disease	Autoimmune disease, hypersensitivity reactions, and nephrotoxicity
Succimer	Lead poisoning	Gastrointestinal distress, rash, CNS effects

[1]Ethylenediaminetetraacetic acid.

    B. Poison Identification
        1. Drug-induced acidosis (anion gap increase) occurs in toxicity from alcohols, aspirin, iron, isoniazid, and verapamil.
        2. Hyperkalemia may be indicative of poisoning from β blockers, digoxin, fluoride, and lithium; **hypokalemia** is caused by overdose of β-adrenoceptor agonists, methylxanthines, and most diuretics.
        3. Many drugs cause characteristic syndromes in overdose (Table 10–3).
    C. Elimination
        1. Gastric lavage with or without activated charcoal may be used for oral ingestion of many drugs.
        2. Alkaline diuresis removes barbiturates, fluoride, and salicylates; **acid diuresis** removes amphetamine, nicotine, and phencyclidine.
        3. Hemodialysis removes many drugs including acetaminophen, alcohols, lithium, quinidine, salicylates, and theophylline.
    D. Antidotes
        1. Specific antidotes exist for only a few poisons.
        2. Table 10–4 lists antidotes for some toxic agents.

ACETAMINOPHEN HEPATOTOXICITY

- *At high doses, when normal pathways of its metabolism are saturated, acetaminophen is converted to a potentially toxic metabolite that is inactivated by glutathione.*
- *If glutathione is depleted (in overdose) the toxic metabolite interacts with liver cells to cause centrilobular necrosis.*
- *Acetylcysteine is antidotal via several mechanisms: it increases glutathione, it inhibits formation of the toxic metabolite, and it can directly interact with the toxic metabolite.*
- *In an adult, hepatotoxicity can occur with ingestion of less than 12 g of acetaminophen, a dose equivalent to 24 normal-strength tablets.*

Table 10–3. Toxic syndromes.

Drug Group	Signs and Symptoms	Interventions
Acetylcholinesterase inhibitors	Diarrhea, urination, miosis, bronchoconstriction, bradycardia, excitation, lacrimation, sweating, salivation (mnemonic: DUMBBELSS)	Support respiration; treat with atropine + pralidoxime; decontaminate
Antimuscarinics	Hyperthermia, dry/hot skin, mydriasis, tachycardia, hypertension, decreased bowel sounds, delirium, seizures	Control hyperthermia; treat with physostigmine
CNS stimulants	Agitation, anxiety, mydriasis, tachycardia, warm/sweaty skin, hypertension, hyperthermia, seizures, increased muscle tone	Control seizures, hypertension, and hyperthermia
Opioids	Sedation, bradycardia, pinpoint pupils, hypotension, hypoventilation, cool skin, flaccid muscles	Airway and respiratory support; treat with naloxone
Salicylates	Confusion, lethargy, hyperventilation, hyperthermia, dehydration, hypokalemia, anion gap acidosis, seizures	Correct acidosis and fluids and electrolytes; increase elimination by alkaline diuresis or hemodialysis
Sedative-hypnotics	Lethargy, nystagmus, decreased muscle tone, hypoventilation, hypothermia, coma	Airway and respiratory support; flumazenil if benzodiazepines are suspected
Tricyclic antidepressants	Antimuscarinic effects (see above), the three "Cs" of coma, convulsions, and cardiotoxicity	Control seizures and hyperthermia, use bicarbonate to correct acidosis and cardiotoxicity

Table 10–4. Specific antidotes.

Antidote	Toxic Agent
Acetylcysteine	Acetaminophen
Atropine + pralidoxime	Acetylcholinesterase inhibitors, including insecticides
Digoxin immune Fab	Digoxin
Ethanol or fomepizole[1]	Ethylene glycol, methanol
Flumazenil	Benzodiazepines, zolpidem, zaleplon
Naloxone	Heroin, morphine, and other opioid analgesics
Oxygen	Carbon monoxide
Physostigmine	Muscarinic blockers
Activated charcoal	Oral poisonings except iron, cyanide, lithium, solvents, acids, corrosives

[1]Inhibits alcohol dehydrogenase.

CLINICAL PROBLEMS

An old pick-up truck with two small children in the enclosed back arrives at a hospital emergency room (ER). According to their father, a farmer, during a 5-hour journey in cold weather the children (who were hitherto quite healthy) had become "sick" with symptoms of gastrointestinal distress, headache, and dizziness. They are now lethargic and have elevated body temperature, and ocular examination reveals bright red retinal veins. The ER physician draws blood for laboratory studies.

1. If these children are suffering from drug or chemical toxicity the most likely causative agent is which of the following?

   A. An organophosphate inhibitor of acetylcholinesterase

   B. Carbon monoxide

   C. Ethylene glycol (antifreeze)

   D. Hydrocyanic acid

   E. Sulfur dioxide

2. Which of the following statements about the poisoning that occurred in these children is accurate?

   A. Cherry-red skin occurs in 80% of patients with this type of poisoning

   B. Inhalation of smoke from fires is the most common cause of this type of poisoning

   C. Management will involve the use of atropine plus pralidoxime

   D. Myocardial ischemia can result from interaction of the toxic compound with myoglobin

   E. Oxygen should not be administered before analysis of serum carboxyhemoglobin levels

3. In the management of a toxic reaction to methylenedioxymethamphetamine (MDMA, "ecstasy") which of the following is least likely to be of clinical value?

   A. Antipyretic drugs to lower body temperature

   B. Benzodiazepine use

   C. Decontamination with activated charcoal

   D. Ice packs

   E. Use of fluids and furosemide if rhabdomyolysis occurs

4. Phencyclidine, a commonly abused drug, is a weakly basic compound. However, urinary acidification is not usually helpful in severe toxicity because of which of the following?

   A. Blood pH is elevated in phencyclidine overdose

   B. In rhabdomyolysis, acidification will increase nephrotoxicity

   C. It interferes with the antiseizure actions of benzodiazepines

   D. Phencyclidine is a quaternary amine

   E. The pK_a of phencyclidine is too low for ionization to occur

5. Regarding acute salicylate poisoning from overdose, which of the following statements is accurate?

   A. Acidification of the urine enhances salicylate elimination

   B. Depression of respiratory drive is an early sign of salicylism

   C. Oral ingestion of 20 mg/kg is associated with severe toxicity

   D. The mortality rate in salicylate poisoning exceeds 5%

   E. Salicylates are effectively eliminated by hemodialysis

A child is brought to an emergency room after ingesting an unknown quantity of a rodenticide. Signs and symptoms include severe gastrointestinal distress, vomiting, and diarrhea with "ricewater" stools. A garlicky odor is detected on the breath.

6. The most likely cause of the toxic syndrome in this child is which of the following?

   A. Arsenic

   B. Cyanide

C. Malathion

D. Paraquat

E. Rotenone

7. Following the ingestion of mushrooms a hungry camper becomes "red as a beet, dry as a bone, and blind as a bat." Supportive treatment should be provided together with the prompt administration of

A. Atropine

B. Flumazenil

C. Naloxone

D. Physostigmine

E. Pralidoxime

A 3-year-old child who ingests a number of prenatal multivitamin tablets prescribed for his mother is brought to the hospital suffering from severe gastroenteritis with bloody diarrhea. Whole bowel irrigation is initiated to flush out unabsorbed pills, and supportive therapy is provided for gastrointestinal bleeding, acidosis, and shock.

8. Which one of the following antidotes should be given systemically to this child?

A. Acetylcysteine

B. Activated charcoal

C. Deferoxamine

D. Fomepizole

E. Succimer

ANSWERS

1. The answer is B. The symptoms and circumstances suggest that the children are suffering from carbon monoxide (CO) poisoning due to inhalation of automobile exhaust. Children journeying in the back of campers or enclosed pick-up trucks are especially vulnerable. Tissue hypoxia occurs because the affinity of CO for hemoglobin (Hb) is over 200 times that of oxygen. Bright red retinal veins on ocular examination are highly suggestive of CO poisoning and confirmation of the diagnosis is made by analysis of serum carboxyhemoglobin (HbCO) (levels > 16% are associated with symptoms).

2. The answer is D. Cherry-red skin is uncommon in CO poisoning; pallor occurs in 80% of poisoned patients. Inhalation of automobile exhaust (accidental or intentional) is the most common cause of CO poisoning. Oxygen (100%) via facemask should be administered immediately if CO poisoning is suspected. The affinity of CO for myoglobin is even greater than that for hemoglobin and may result in myocardial ischemia.

3. The answer is A. MDMA toxicity has characteristics similar to those of amphetamine-like CNS stimulants and hyperthermia is a common feature. Ice packs should be applied, but antipyretic drugs do not reduce hyperthermia caused by MDMA overdose. Gastric lavage with activated charcoal may be helpful if ingestion of the drug is recent. Benzodiazepines may reduce anxiety and muscle cramps and would be used if seizures occur. Adequate fluids, with the use of diuretics, help protect renal function in rhabdomyolysis.

4. The answer is B. In principle, urinary acidification should increase the ionization state of weak bases and accelerate their renal elimination. However, in cases of toxicity due to CNS stimulants that may cause damage to skeletal muscles (eg, amphetamine and phencyclidine) the kidney must be protected by use of fluids, diuretics, and alkalinization. The pK_a of phencyclidine is > 8. Quaternary amines do not cross the blood–brain barrier.

5. The answer is E. Alkalinization of the urine increases the renal clearance of salicylate, a weak acid. Stimulation of the respiratory center leads to hyperventilation, an early sign of salicylate toxicity. The dose of aspirin associated with severe toxicity is over 200 mg/kg, which in a 70-kg patient is approximately 40 regular-strength tablets. In 1998 over 14,000 aspirin poisonings were reported to poison control centers in the United States, resulting in 33 deaths—a mortality rate of < 0.3%.

6. The answer is A. Most accidental poisoning due to arsenic occurs in an industrial setting. However, arsenic used in rodenticides and in wood preservatives sometimes causes toxicity following the ingestion of such products. Acute poisoning results in the described symptoms plus severe dehydration, electrolyte imbalance, and shock. Gastric decontamination, supportive care, and chelation therapy are the mainstays of management.

7. The answer is D. The classic anticholinergic syndrome includes flushed skin, dry mucous membranes, hyperthermia, blurred vision, confusion, and delirium. Pupils are dilated, skeletal muscles twitch, and patients usually have sinus tachycardia. A variety of plants and fungi contain atropinelike compounds and many drugs used for other purposes (eg, antihistamines and tricyclic antidepressants) also have anticholinergic effects. The specific antidote for peripheral and central anticholinergic syndrome is physostigmine.

8. The answer is C. The child is suffering from acute iron poisoning and deferoxamine, an iron chelator, should be administered. Activated charcoal, an effective absorbent for many toxins, does not bind iron. Can you identify the other antidotes listed?

CHAPTER 11
SPECIAL TOPICS

I. Gastrointestinal Pharmacology

A. Drugs used in acid-peptic disease include **H$_2$-receptor blockers, proton pump inhibitors, mucosal protective agents,** and **antacids** (Figure 11–1); antibiotics are important drugs for the eradication of *Helicobacter pylori,* the causative agent in most patients with peptic ulcers.

1. The H$_2$ blockers (**cimetidine** and others) are very effective in controlling symptoms of uncomplicated peptic ulcer, but are less effective in Zollinger-Ellison syndrome with hypergastrinemia and in gastroesophageal reflux disease (GERD).
   a. They are relatively safe and are available over the counter, although cimetidine is a cytochrome P-450 (CYP450) enzyme inhibitor and may inhibit metabolism of other drugs (see Table 11–5).
   b. Other H$_2$ blockers do not inhibit CYP450.

2. The proton pump inhibitors (**omeprazole** and others) are the most efficacious agents available for reducing acid secretion.
   a. They irreversibly inhibit the H$^+$,K$^+$-ATPase in gastric parietal cells and thus can reduce acid secretion to negligible values for 24–48 hours.
   b. They are heavily used in GERD and in the much less common Zollinger-Ellison syndrome.
   c. They are reasonably safe and have been proposed for over-the-counter use.

3. Mucosal protective agents include the prostaglandin E$_1$ analog **misoprostol,** and **sucralfate.**
   a. In the acid environment of the stomach, sucralfate polymerizes to form a protective coating over the ulcer bed.
   b. It is essentially free of systemic toxicity because it is not absorbed.

4. Antacids are weak bases that chemically neutralize acid.
   a. The most commonly used include **aluminum hydroxide, magnesium hydroxide,** and combinations of the two.
   b. They are less effective than the other agents listed above.

ANTIBIOTICS IN PEPTIC ULCER

- *The eradication of* Helicobacter pylori *with the use of antibiotics has contributed significantly to the successful treatment of peptic ulcer disease.*
- *Antibiotics used in combinations with antacids (H$_2$ blockers or proton pump inhibitors) include **amoxicillin, clarithromycin, metronidazole,** and **tetracycline.***

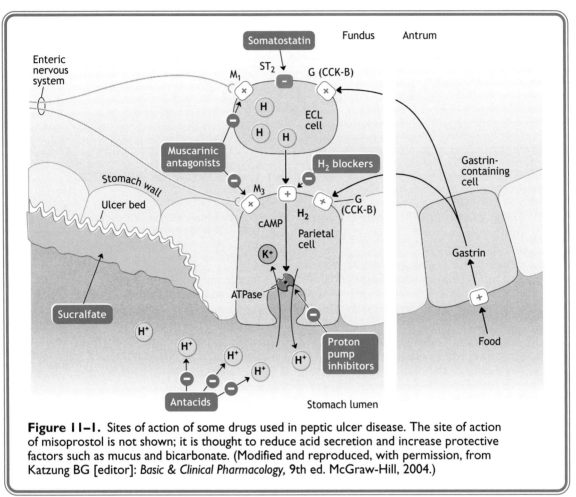

Figure 11–1. Sites of action of some drugs used in peptic ulcer disease. The site of action of misoprostol is not shown; it is thought to reduce acid secretion and increase protective factors such as mucus and bicarbonate. (Modified and reproduced, with permission, from Katzung BG [editor]: *Basic & Clinical Pharmacology,* 9th ed. McGraw-Hill, 2004.)

B. **Gastroparesis** is a loss of esophageal and gastric emptying motility that occurs in patients with diabetes and other diseases associated with damage to visceral nerves.
   1. Gastroparesis causes severe bloating, pain, and sometimes vomiting.
   2. Gastric motility can be stimulated with **metoclopramide,** a dopamine antagonist and releaser of acetylcholine (ACh) in the gut, and by **cisapride,** a 5-hydroxytryptamine (5-HT$_4$, serotonin) agonist.
   3. Metoclopramide enters the central nervous system (CNS) and may cause parkinsonian symptoms.
   4. Cisapride causes prolongation of the QT interval and has been restricted because of fatal arrhythmias.
C. **Antiemetic drugs** are extremely important for the control of nausea and vomiting caused by cancer chemotherapy and surgical anesthesia. Representative agents and proposed mechanisms are given in Table 11–1.

Table 11–1. Antiemetic drugs.

Drug	Class and Proposed Mechanism	Comments
Ondansetron	5-HT$_3$ antagonist	High efficacy, widely used
Dexamethasone	Corticosteroid, unknown	Moderate efficacy, widely used
Diphenhydramine	H$_1$ blocker	Moderate to low efficacy
Metoclopramide	Dopamine antagonist	Moderate to low efficacy
Prochlorperazine	Dopamine antagonist	Moderate efficacy also in motion sickness
Dronabinol	Cannabinoid, unknown	Moderate to low efficacy

    D. Laxatives act by several mechanisms: irritation of the bowel (**castor oil** and **senna**), bulk formation (**magnesium hydroxide** and **psyllium**), stool softening (**docusate**), and lubrication (**mineral oil** and **glycerine**).

    E. Antidiarrheal drugs include opioid derivatives that act on mu opioid receptors in the gut. The most important are **loperamide, diphenoxylate,** and **difenoxin** (the active metabolite of diphenoxylate).

II. Vaccines and Other Immunization Materials

    A. Passive immunization uses preformed antibodies (usually **immunoglobulins**) from human or animal sources to transfer immunity to the host.

        1. Animal antibodies may cause hypersensitivity reactions.

        2. Human **immune globulin** is used in organ and tissue transplantation, in hypogammaglobulinemia, and for prevention of hepatitis A infection postexposure.

        3. Other **antiviral products** include immune globulins against cytomegalovirus, hepatitis B, rabies, respiratory syncytial virus, vaccinia, and varicella.

        4. Antibacterial products include botulism antitoxin and tetanus immune globulin.

        5. Rh$_o$(D) immune globulin is used in Rh-negative women to prevent hemolytic disease of the newborn.

        6. Passive immunization includes the use of **antivenins** for treatment of black widow spider bites and snake bites (eg, coral and crotalid snakes).

    B. In **active immunization,** antigens, which stimulate antibody formation and host cell-mediated immunity, are used to confer long-lasting immunity against disease vectors.

        1. Live (attenuated) immunogens include vaccines for measles, mumps, poliovirus, rubella, and varicella.

        2. Products using **dead immunogens** include *Haemophilus influenzae* type B conjugates (Hib conjugates), inactivated hepatitis A and B and influenza viral antigens, rabies vaccine, and tetanus-diphtheria toxoids (Td).

3. Bacterial polysaccharide vaccines are used for active immunization of persons at high risk of infection from meningococci and pneumococci; a recombinant bacterial protein is used to prevent Lyme disease.

VACCINATION WITH *HAEMOPHILUS INFLUENZAE* TYPE B CONJUGATE

CLINICAL
CORRELATION

- *Vaccination against invasive diseases caused by* Haemophilus influenzae *type B in children at the age of 2 months became available in the United States in 1990.*
- *In the past decade the epidemiology of infection has changed dramatically because of the widespread use of Hib conjugate vaccines.*
- *In populations with high rates of vaccination, the incidence of disease due to* Haemophilus influenzae *type B has decreased by more than 95%.*
- *Vaccination decreases nasopharyngeal carriage and the spread of infection, thus even unimmunized children may be protected.*

   C. A schedule for **active immunization of children** is given in Table 11–2.

III. Botanicals and Nutritional Supplements

   A. Concepts
   1. **Botanicals** (**herbals**) and **nutritional supplements** are marketed without Food and Drug Administration (FDA) review of efficacy or safety.
   2. No requirements exist regarding the purity, potency, or chemical composition of such products.
   3. In many cases evidence for medical effectiveness is incomplete or nonexistent.

Table 11–2. Schedule for active immunization of children.

Age	Material Administered
Birth	HBV (hepatitis B vaccine)
2 months	DTap (toxoids of diphtheria and tetanus, acellular pertussis vaccine); IPV (inactivated polio vaccine); Hib (Haemophilus influenzae type B conjugate); HBV; PCV (pneumococcal conjugate vaccine)
4 months	DTap; IPV; Hib; PCV
6 months	DTap; Hib; PCV
6–18 months	IPV; HBV; influenza, split virius vaccine
12–18 months	DTap; Hib; MMR (measles, mumps, and rubella vaccine); varicella vaccine
4–6 years	DTap; IPV; MMR
11–12 years	Td (tetanus–diphtheria toxoids)

Table 11–3. Possible uses and important toxicities of "natural" medicinals.

Agent	Clinical Uses	Toxicities
Echinacea	Common cold	Gastrointestinal distress, dizziness, and headache
Ephedra	As for ephedrine	CNS and cardiovascular stimulation; arrhythmias, stroke, and seizures at high doses
Feverfew	Migraine	Gastrointestinal distress, mouth ulcers, and antiplatelet actions
Ginkgo	Intermittent claudication	Gastrointestinal distress, anxiety, insomnia, headache, and antiplatelet actions
Kava	Chronic anxiety	Gastrointestinal distress, sedation, ataxia, hepatotoxicity, phototoxicity, and dermatotoxicity
Milk thistle	Viral hepatitis	Loose stools
Saw palmetto	Benign prostatic hyperplasia	Gastrointestinal distress, decreased libido, and hypertension
St. John's wort	Mild–moderate depression	Gastrointestinal distress and phototoxicity; serotonin syndrome with SSRIs; induces cytochrome P-450 enzymes
Dehydroepiandrosterone	Symptomatic improvement in females with SLE or AIDS	Androgenization (premenopausal women), estrogenic effects (postmenopausal), and feminization (young men)
Melatonin	Jet lag, insomnia	Sedation, suppresses mid-cycle luteinizing hormone, and hypoprolactinemia

B. Possible Clinical Uses
  1. Conditions for which clinical trials of botanicals or nutritional supplements have suggested possible effectiveness are shown in Table 11–3.
  2. Table 11–3 also lists common toxicities of these agents.

EPHEDRA

- *Extracts of plants from the genus* Ephedra *(eg, ma-huang) contain ephedrine and pseudoephedrine.*
- *Prior to recent FDA regulations, ephedra products were commonly used for respiratory disorders such as asthma and bronchitis, as nasal decongestants, and as aids to weight reduction.*
- *In Chinese medicine, ma-huang is used for relief of cold and flu symptoms, for diuresis, and for bone and joint pain.*
- *Cardiotoxicity is a major problem in overdose.*

CLINICAL CORRELATION

Table 11–4. Claimed uses and important toxicities of selected botanicals.

Agent	Intended Uses	Toxicities
Aconite	Analgesic (topical and oral)	Cardiac and CNS toxicity with oral use
Borage	Anti-inflammatory, diuretic	Gastrointestinal distress and hepatic dysfunction with oral use
Chaparral	Anti-infective, antioxidant	Hepatic and renal dysfunction
Coltsfoot	Anti-infective	Allergies, phototoxicity, and hepatic dysfunction
Germander	Dietary and digestive aid	Hepatitis and complete liver failure
Jimsonweed	Respiratory tract diseases	Atropinelike CNS and peripheral toxicities
Pennyroyal	Abortifacient, induces menses, digestive aid	CNS dysfunction, hematemesis, liver and renal dysfunction, disseminated intra-vascular coagulation
Pokeweed	Root extracts for emesis and rheumatism	Bloody diarrhea, hypotension, respiratory failure, coma, and blindness
Royal jelly	Immune potentiation, tonic, hyperlipidemias	Allergic reactions including anaphylaxis
Sassafras	Anticoagulant, urinary tract disorders; oil used topically as antiseptic	Diaphoresis and hot flushes with use of bark; ingestion of oil may cause cardiovascular and respiratory collapse

• Contraindications are the same as those for ephedrine and include anxiety states, cardiac arrhythmias, diabetes, glaucoma, heart failure, hypertension, hyperthyroidism, and pregnancy.

    C. **Claimed Clinical Uses**
        1. Conditions for which botanicals have not yet been proven effective are shown in Table 11–4.
        2. Table 11–4 also lists common toxicities of these agents.
    D. **Botanical–Drug Interactions**
        1. Garlic and **ginkgo** increase the risk of bleeding when used with anticoagulant or antiplatelet drugs.

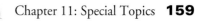

2. Additive CNS depression occurs if **kava** is used with sedative-hypnotics including alcohol.

3. **Ma-huang** and **ephedra** products are additive with sympathomimetics.

4. **St. John's wort** may increase the effects of antidepressant drugs and decrease the effectiveness of cyclosporine, indinavir, oral contraceptives, and warfarin.

IV. Drug Interactions

A. Concepts

1. **Drug interactions** involve changes in the duration or intensity of a drug's action caused by the presence of another drug.

2. **Pharmacokinetic factors** include interactions at the level of drug absorption, distribution, metabolism, and excretion.

3. **Pharmacodynamic factors** include drug interactions based on opposing effects or additive actions.

DRUG INTERACTIONS WITH WARFARIN

CLINICAL CORRELATION

- *The anticoagulant effects of warfarin are increased by drugs that inhibit its metabolism, including cimetidine, erythromycin, ketoconazole, and lovastatin.*
- *Pharmacodynamic actions can also contribute to enhanced anticoagulant effects when warfarin is used concomitantly with anabolic steroids, aspirin, nonsteroidal anti-inflammatory drugs (NSAIDs), and thyroxine.*
- *Drugs that induce enzymes responsible for the metabolism of warfarin (eg, barbiturates, carbamazepine, phenytoin, and rifampin) may decrease its anticoagulant effects by facilitating its clearance from the body.*

B. Pharmacokinetic Drug Interactions

1. Drugs that enhance the effects of other agents by inhibiting their metabolism by the major form of cytochrome P-450 (3A4) include amiodarone, cimetidine, ciprofloxacin, erythromycin, fluvoxamine, indinavir, ketoconazole, ritonavir, and venlafaxine.

2. Drugs that decrease the effects of other agents by inducing the activity of cytochrome P-450 enzymes include barbiturates, carbamazepine, ethanol, glucocorticoids, phenytoin, and rifampin.

3. Representative pharmacokinetic interactions of clinical significance are shown in Table 11–5.

C. Pharmacodynamic Drug Interactions

1. One of the most frequent drug interactions of this type is additive CNS depression when drugs from the following groups are used in combinations with each other: alcohols, anesthetics, most anticonvulsants, antipsychotics, strong opioid analgesics, sedative-hypnotics, and tricyclic antidepressants.

2. Representative pharmacodynamic interactions of clinical significance are shown in Table 11–6.

Table 11–5. Important pharmacokinetic drug interactions.

Drug or Drug Group	Drug(s) Affected	Comment
Antacids	Fluoroquinolones, keto-conazole, tetracyclines	Interference with oral absorption
Antibiotics	Oral contraceptives	Increased clearance of estrogens
Bile acid sequestrants	Acetaminophen, digoxin, thiazides, warfarin	Interference with oral absorption
Carbamazepine	Estrogens, haloperidol, theophylline, warfarin	Increased clearance due to induction of drug-metabolizing enzymes
Cimetidine	Benzodiazepines, lidocaine, phenytoin, quinidine, warfarin	Decreased clearance due to inhibition of drug-metabolizing enzymes
Erythromycin	Cisapride, quinidine, sildenafil, theophylline	Decreased clearance due to inhibition of drug-metabolizing enzymes
Ketoconazole	Cyclosporine, fluoxetine, lovastatin, quinidine, warfarin	Decreased clearance due to inhibition of drug-metabolizing enzymes
Monoamine oxidase (MAO) inhibitors	Indirect-acting sympathomimetics and tyramine-containing foods	Increased amounts of norepinephrine released from sympathetic nerve endings
Phenytoin	Methadone, quinidine, steroids, verapamil	Increased clearance due to induction of drug-metabolizing enzymes
Rifampin	Azoles, methadone, steroids, theophylline	Increased clearance due to induction of drug-metabolizing enzymes
Ritonavir	Antidepressants, carba-mazepine, dronabinol, ondansetron, triazolam	Decreased clearance due to inhibition of drug-metabolizing enzymes

CLINICAL PROBLEMS

A 32-year-old female executive presents at a gastrointestinal clinic for follow-up after recovering from a bleeding duodenal ulcer.

Table 11–6. Important pharmacodynamic drug interactions.

Drug or Drug Group	Drug(s) Affected	Comment
Alcohol	Anesthetics, anticonvulsants, and sedative-hypnotics	Additive CNS depression
	Cephalosporins and metronidazole	Disulfiramlike reactions via alde- hyde dehydrogenase inhibition
Aminoglycosides	Loop diuretics	Enhanced ototoxicity
Antihistaminics	Antimuscarinics and sedatives	Enhanced anticholinergic and CNS depressant effects
β Blockers	Insulin and sulfonylureas	Mask hypoglycemic symptoms
	α-Adrenoceptor blockers	Increased "first-dose" syncope
Nonsteroidal anti-inflammatory drugs (NSAIDs)	Angiotensin-converting enzyme (ACE) inhibitors and diuretics	Decreased effectiveness of ACE inhibitors and diuretics
Salicylates	Glucocorticoids	Increased GI toxicity with steroids
	Sulfinpyrazone	Decreased effects of uricosurics
Selective sero- tonin reuptake inhibitors (SSRIs)	MAO inhibitors, tricyclic antidepressants	Increased risk of serotonin syndrome
Warfarin	Antiplatelet drugs, heparins, NSAIDs	Enhanced bleeding

1. Which of the following statements is most accurate?

    A. Because of teratogenicity, use of omeprazole in this woman is contraindicated unless she uses at least two methods of contraception

    B. Use of misoprostol is likely to be complicated by constipation

    C. Cimetidine therapy may result in interactions with other drugs

    D. Sucralfate is convenient but is often associated with sedation

    E. Oral antacid therapy is the most convenient and inexpensive effective follow-up therapy

A 25-year-old man is to be treated with intensive chemotherapy for Hodgkin's lymphoma. Because of the risk of drug-induced emesis, an antiemetic regimen is proposed.

2. Which of the following is the **least** likely to be selected?

    A. Metoclopramide, dronabinol, diphenhydramine

    B. Ondansetron, metoclopramide, diphenhydramine

C. Dexamethasone, ondansetron, diphenhydramine

    D. Prochlorperazine, dexamethasone, ondansetron, diphenhydramine

    E. Diphenhydramine, dexamethasone, ondansetron, metoclopramide

While gardening, a young woman is bitten by a rattlesnake and serious envenomation en-
sues. When hospitalized her treatment involves passive immunization using antivenin.

3. Which of the following statements about the care of this patient is accurate?

    A. Antivenin does not cause hypersensitivity since it is of human origin

    B. Live (attenuated) immunogens are used in passive immunization

    C. Palivizumab is now available for treatment of envenomation caused by all cro-
       talid snakes

    D. Serum sickness from antivenin occurs commonly follows its use in serious en-
       venomation from rattlesnake bites

    E. Treatment with human immune globulin is the standard of care in snake bites

4. An "active–passive" immunization approach may be used in the treatment of health
care workers following needlestick accidents to protect against infection due to which
of the following?

    A. Cytomegalovirus

    B. Hepatitis B virus

    C. Human immunodeficiency virus

    D. Herpes simplex virus

    E. Varicella zoster

Highly active antiretroviral therapy (HAART) with zidovudine, lamivudine, and ritonavir
has reversed the decline in $CD4^+$ cells in an AIDS patient, and his viral RNA load has decreased during the past 2 months of treatment. The patient is also prescribed carbamazepine for neuropathic pain, dronabinol to stimulate appetite, ketoconazole for
prophylaxis against oral candidiasis, ondansetron for emesis, fluoxetine for depression, and
triazolam for insomnia. He takes over-the-counter ranitidine for indigestion and ibuprofen for headaches.

5. Which of the following pairs of drugs is most likely to enhance the actions of the other
drugs that the patient is taking?

    A. Carbamazepine and triazolam

    B. Dronabinol and fluoxetine

    C. Ketoconazole and ritonavir

    D. Ondansetron and ibuprofen

    E. Ranitidine and carbamazepine

6. A drug interaction resulting from consumption of alcoholic beverages is **least** likely to
occur in a patient being treated with which of the following?

    A. Amitriptyline for depression

    B. Buspirone for chronic anxiety

C. Cefotetan for pelvic inflammatory disease

   D. Diphenhydramine for allergic rhinitis

   E. Methadone for severe pain

The proposed clinical benefits of many botanicals and nutritional supplements are often only weakly substantiated by controlled studies.

7. Which of the following pairs of agent: established use is best documented?

   A. Dehydroepiandrosterone (DHEA): benign prostatic hyperplasia

   B. Echinacea: migraine

   C. Ephedra: paroxysmal supraventricular tachycardia

   D. Melatonin: jet lag

   E. St. John's wort: Alzheimer's disease

8. Which of the following effects is common to both feverfew and ginkgo?

   A. Antiplatelet actions

   B. Decreased libido

   C. Hepatotoxicity

   D. Migraine

   E. Phototoxicity

ANSWERS

1. The answer is C. Cimetidine, an H_2-receptor blocker, is a potent inhibitor of cytochrome P-450 drug-metabolizing enzymes and has been associated with decreased clearance of benzodiazepines, phenytoin, warfarin, and other drugs. Other H_2 blockers are not associated with P-450 inhibition. Omeprazole is not associated with teratogenic effects, although gastrointestinal tumors have been observed in rats treated with very high doses. Misoprostol commonly causes diarrhea. Sucralfate is not absorbed and causes no systemic effects. Antacids must be taken several times daily in large doses; they are not convenient and are thus unpopular except for over-the-counter treatment of mild gastroesophageal reflux.

2. The answer is A. Almost all regimens for chemotherapy-induced vomiting include ondansetron or another $5\text{-}HT_3$ antagonist (granisetron or dolasetron) because these are the most efficacious and least toxic antiemetics currently available. All the other drugs listed are often included in such regimens and four-drug and five-drug "cocktails" are common.

3. The answer is D. Crotalid antivenin is equine-derived and serum sickness invariably occurs when it is used to treat serious envenomation. Immune globulin is ineffective in snake bites, but is widely used for passive immunization in organ and tissue transplantation. Palivizumab is a monoclonal antibody that is protective against respiratory syncytial virus. Live (attenuated) and dead immunogens are used in active immunization.

4. The answer is B. Needlestick injury from a patient with hepatitis B surface antigen (HbsAg)-positive blood requires that both the vaccine (recombinant inactive viral antigen) and hepatitis B immune globulin (HBIG) be administered at separate sites. The vaccine provides long-term protection (active immunization), whereas HBIG provides immediate protection (passive immunization).

5. The answer is C. Ketoconazole and ritonavir inhibit hepatic cytochrome P-450 isozymes, enhancing the actions of many drugs including dronabinol, fluoxetine, ondansetron, and triazolam. Ranitidine is much less likely to inhibit drug metabolism than its congener cimetidine. Fluoxetine is reported to inhibit a specific P-450 isozyme, but none of the drugs taken by the AIDS patient described in this case is a substrate for that enzyme.

6. The answer is B. The most common drug interactions involving ethanol are pharmacodynamic, resulting in additive depression of CNS functions when used in patients taking drugs that have sedative actions. Such drugs include sedative-hypnotics, strong opioid analgesics, tricyclic antidepressants, and over-the-counter antihistamines (eg, diphenhydramine). Cefotetan inhibits aldehyde dehydrogenase and may cause disulfiramlike reactions with ethanol. Buspirone, a selective nonsedating anxiolytic, does not cause additive CNS depression with ethanol.

7. The answer is D. In older men DHEA increases androgen synthesis and should be avoided in patients with benign prostatic hyperplasia (BPH); saw palmetto may improve symptoms in some BPH patients. Although echinacea may reduce symptoms of the common cold, it is not used in migraine; feverfew is the herbal that appears to be of some value in migraine. The risk of cardiotoxicity from products containing ephedra precludes their use in persons with a history of arrhythmias or hypertension. St. John's wort may have value in mild to moderate depression, but unlike DHEA and ginkgo products, it has not been claimed to have useful effects in Alzheimer's disease.

8. The answer is A. Both feverfew and ginkgo have antiplatelet actions that may increase bleeding liability in patients maintained on anticoagulants. Feverfew is effective in migraine in some patients; ginkgo has been used to treat "cerebral insufficiency" in Alzheimer's disease. Saw palmetto inhibits 5α-reductase and its use in benign prostatic hyperplasia may result in decreased libido. Botanicals associated with hepatotoxicity include borage, chaparral, coltsfoot, germander, and pennyroyal. Phototoxicity is an adverse effect of coltsfoot, kava, and St. John's wort.

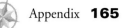

Table A–1. Major drug groups and their most important members.

Drug Group (Chapter Number)	Most Important Members
Androgens and antiandrogrens (6)	Androgens (methyltestosterone, oxandrolone); receptor antagonists (flutamide); 5α-reductase inhibitors (finasteride); synthesis inhibitors (ketoconazole); gonadotropin-releasing hormone (GnRH) analogs (leuprolide)
Anemia drugs (4)	Iron (ferrous sulfate, ferrous gluconate, iron dextran); folic acid; cyanocobalamin (vitamin B_{12}); epoetin; filgrastim (granulo-cyte colony-stimulating factor, G-CSF), sargramostim (granulo-cyte-macrophage colony-stimulating factor, GM-CSF)
Anesthetics (5)	Inhaled (halothane, isoflurane, nitrous oxide); intravenous (fentanyl, ketamine, midazolam, propofol, thiopental); local anesthetics (procaine, lidocaine)
Antiangina drugs (3)	Nitrates (nitroglycerin, isosorbide dinitrate); β blockers propranolol); calcium channel blockers (nifedipine)
Antiarrhythmics (3)	Sodium channel blockers (lidocaine); sodium + potassium chan-nel blockers (quinidine, procainamide, amiodarone, flecainide); potassium channel blockers (ibutilide, dofetilide); potassium channel + β blockers (sotalol); calcium channel blockers (vera-pamil, diltiazem); I_{K1} activator (adenosine)
Antibacterial drugs (7)	Aminoglycosides (gentamicin); cephalosporins (cefoxitin, cefaclor, ceftriaxone); fluoroquinolones (ciprofloxacin); macrolides (erthromycin, azithromycin); metronidazole; peni-cillins (penicillin G, amoxicillin, ampicillin, nafcillin); tetracyclines (doxycycline); vancomycin Antitubercular drugs (isoniazid, rifampin, ethambutol, pyrazinamide, streptomycin)
Anticancer drugs (9)	Alkylators (cisplatin, cyclophosphamide); antimetabolites (fluorouracil, methotrexate, mercaptopurine); antibiotics (bleomycin, doxorubicin); plant alkaloids (vinblastine, vin-cristine); monoclonal antibodies (trastuzumab)
Antidepressants (5)	Monoamine oxidase (MAO) inhibitors (phenelzine); tricyclics (amitriptyline, imipramine); selective serotonin reuptake inhibitors (SSRIs) (fluoxetine, paroxetine); miscellaneous (bupropion, mirtazapine, trazodone)
Antifungals (8)	Polyenes (amphotericin B, nystatin); azoles (ketoconazole, fluconazole); antimetabolite (flucytosine); antidermatophytics (griseofluvin, terbinafine)

(continued)

Table A–1. Major drug groups and their most important members. (*Continued*)

Drug Group (Chapter Number)	Most Important Members
Antihistamines (4)	
H₁ blockers used for hay fever, urticaria	H₁ blockers; older first generation [H₁ + autonomic nervous system (ANS) block, sedating: diphenhydramine, dimenhydrinate]; newer first generation (less ANS block: chlorpheniramine); second generation (little ANS or sedative effect: loratadine, fexofenadine)
H₂ blockers used for acid-peptic disease	H₂ blockers: cimetidine, ranitidine
Antihypertensives (3)	Diuretics (furosemide, hydrochlorothiazide); sympatholytics (clonidine, reserpine, prazosin, propranolol); vasodilators (hydralazine, minoxidil, calcium channel blockers); angiotensin antagonists [angiotensin-converting enzyme (ACE) inhibitors (captopril, "-prils"); angiotensin receptor blockers (losartan, "-artans")]
Antiparasitics (8)	Antimalarial drugs (chloroquine, mefloquine, primaquine, quinine) Other antiprotozoal drugs (metronidazole, pentamidine, trimethoprim-sulfamethoxazole) Anthelmintics (albendazole, niclosamide, praziquantel, pyrantel pamoate)
Antiplatelet, anticoagulant, thrombolytics, and antilipid drugs (4)	Antiplatelets (aspirin, tirofiban, ticlopidine, clopidogrel, abciximab) Anticoagulants [warfarin, heparin (high- and low-molecular-weight forms)] Thrombolytics (streptokinase, alteplase) Antilipid drugs [niacin, cholestyramine, lovastatin (statins), gemfibrozil (fibrates, ezetimibe)]
Antipsychotics and drugs for bipolar disorder (5)	Atypical antipsychotics (clozapine, olanzapine, risperidone); butyrophenones (haloperidol); phenothiazines (chlorpromazine, fluphenazine, thioridazine) Bipolar disorder drugs (lithium, carbamazepine, clonazepam, gabapentin, valproic acid)
Antiseizure drugs (5)	Older agents (carbamazepine, clonazepam, ethosuximide, phenobarbital, phenytoin, valproic acid) Newer drugs (felbamate, gabapentin, lamotrigine, topiramate)
Antiviral drugs (8)	Antiherpetics (acyclovir, foscarnet, ganciclovir); protease inhibitors (indinavir, ritonavir); reverse transcriptase inhibitors (didanosine, lamivudine, zidovudine); anti-influenzal agents (amantadine, zanamivir); miscellaneous (ribavirin)

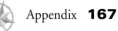

Table A–1. Major drug groups and their most important members. (*Continued*)

Drug Group (Chapter Number)	Most Important Members
Bone mineral drugs (6)	Vitamin D (calcitriol, etc); calcitonin; bisphosphonates (etidronate, alendronate); fluoride; estrogens
Cholinomimetic and anticholinergics (2)	Direct-acting mimetics (bethanechol, pilocarpine, nicotine, succinylcholine) Indirect-acting mimetics (neostigmine, physostigmine, malathion, parathion) Antimuscarinics (atropine, scopolamine, glycopyrrolate) Antinicotinics (hexamethonium, tubocurarine)
Corticosteroids and antagonist drugs (6)	Glucocorticoids (cortisol, prednisone, triamcinolone, dexamethasone); mineralocorticoid (fludrocortisone); glucocorticoid antagonist (mifepristone); mineralocorticoid antagonist (spironolactone); synthesis inhibitors (ketoconazole)
Digitalis and other heart failure (HF) drugs (3)	Digoxin; β_1 agonists (dobutamine); vasodilators; ACE inhibitors and angiotensin antagonists; β blockers; diuretics
Diuretics (3)	Carbonic anhydrase inhibitors (acetazolamide); loop agents (furosemide); thiazides (hydrochlorothiazide); potassium-sparing agents (spironolactone, amiloride); osmotic agents (mannitol)
Drugs acting on 5-hydroxytryptamine (5-HT) receptors (4)	Sumatriptan (5-HT_{1d} agonist); ergot alkaloids (5-HT, α, and dopamine partial agonists); ketanserin (5-HT_2 and α blocker); ondansetron ("-setrons") 5-HT_3 antagonists; cisapride (5-HT_4 agonist)
Drugs for Parkinson's disease (5)	Dopamine (DA) agonists (bromocriptine, pramipexole, ropinirole); DA precursor (levodopa); dopa decarboxylase inhibitor (carbidopa); MAO B inhibitor (selegiline); catechol-O-methyltransferase (COMT) inhibitors (tolcapone); muscarinic blockers (benztropine)
Estrogens and antiestrogens (6)	Estrogens (conjugated equine, ethinyl estradiol, mestranol); partial agonist (clomiphene); selective estrogen receptor modulators (raloxifene, tamoxifen); aromatase inhibitors (anastrozole)
Immune modulators (9)	Immunosuppressants: antibiotics (cyclosporine, tacrolimus); anti–tumor necrosis factor (TNF) (etanercept); antibodies (immune globulins, $Rh_o(D)$ immune globulin); cytotoxics (azathioprine); enzyme inhibitors (mycophenolate mofetil, leflunomide); monoclonal antibodies (abciximab, daclizumab, infliximab) Immunostimulants (aldesleukin, interferons)

(continued)

Table A–1. Major drug groups and their most important members. (*Continued*)

Drug Group (Chapter Number)	Most Important Members
Insulins and oral hypoglycemics (6)	Insulins (lispro, regular, lente, glargine); biguanide (metformin); meglitinide (repaglinide); sulfonylureas (glyburide, glipizide); thiazolidinediones (pioglitazone)
Nonsteroidal anti-inflammatory drugs (NSAIDs), antigout, and antipyretics (4)	NSAIDs (aspirin, salicylate, ibuprofen, indomethacin, many others) Slow-acting antirheumatic drugs (methotrexate, chloroquine, leflunomide, infliximab, etanercept) Antigout (NSAIDs, colchicine, probenecid, allopurinol) Antipyretic analgesic (acetaminophen)
Opioids (5)	Strong agonists (meperidine, methadone, morphine) Moderate agonists (codeine, oxycodone) Antagonists (naloxone, naltrexone) Mixed agonist–antagonists (nalbuphine, pentazocine)
Pituitary–hypothalamus drugs (6)	Growth hormone (GH) agonist (somatropin); GH antagonist (octreotide); ACTH analog (cosyntropin); GnRH partial agonists (leuprolide); follicle-stimulating hormone (FSH) analog (urofollitropin); luteinizing hormone (LH) analog [human chorionic gonadotropin (hCG)]; vasopressin (antidiuretic hormone, ADH); desmopressin (ADH analog)
Progestins and antiprogestins (6)	Progestins (medroxyprogesterone, norgestrel, norethindrone); partial agonist (danazol); antagonist (mifepristone)
Prostaglandins and nitric oxide (4)	Alprostadil, misoprostol (PGE_1 analogs); latanoprost ($PGF_{2\alpha}$ analog); epoprostenol (PGI_2); nitric oxide gas
Sedatives and hypnotics (5)	Alcohols (chloral hydrate, ethanol); barbiturates (pentobarbital, phenobarbital); benzodiazepines (alprazolam, diazepam, triazolam); buspirone; zolpidem
Sympathomimetics and sympatholytics (2)	Direct-acting agonists (norepinephrine, epinephrine, isoproterenol, albuterol, phenylephrine) Indirect-acting agonists (amphetamine, ephedrine, cocaine) α Antagonists [phenoxybenzamine, phentolamine, prazosin ("-osins")] β Blockers (propranolol, atenolol, metoprolol, pindolol, labetalol)
Thyroid and anti-thyroid drugs (6)	Thyroxine, triiodothyronine Antithyroid [propylthiouracil, iodide, ipodate, radioactive iodine (^{131}I)]

(continued)

Table A–2. Drugs to avoid in pregnancy.

Pregnancy Risk Categories[1]	Description of Risk	Drugs to Avoid
X	Unsafe; absolutely contraindicated	Acitretin, clomiphene, cocaine (as illicit drug), ergots, ethanol, HMG-CoA reductase inhibitors, isotretinoin, misoprostol, nicotine, Premarin (conjugated equine estrogens), quinine, raloxifene, ribavirin, thalidomide
D	Evidence of risk, but in certain circumstances use may be justifiable	ACE inhibitors and angiotensin antagonists (second and third trimesters), aminoglycosides, amiodarone, atenolol, benzodiazepines, cytotoxic anticancer drugs and immunosuppressants, lithium, phenytoin, tetracyclines, valproic acid, warfarin
C	Uncertain safety; animal studies demonstrate effects on fetal development	ACE inhibitors and angiotensin antagonists (first trimester), carbamazepine, clarithromycin, fluoroquinolones, NSAIDs (near term)

[1]Most category C drugs listed above are not approved by the FDA for use in pregnancy.

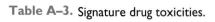

Table A–3. Signature drug toxicities.

Toxicity	Drug or Drug Groups
Agranulocytosis	Clozapine, chloramphenicol, gold salts, indomethacin, propylthiouracil, methimazole
Atropinelike effects	Antihistaminics, clozapine, thioridazine, tricyclic antidepressants
Cardiotoxicity (most drugs used for cardio-vascular disorders are potentially cardiotoxic)	Doxorubicin, daunorubicin, emetine, fluoroquinolones, glucagon, lithium, tricyclic antidepressants, thioridazine, theophylline
Gingival hyperplasia	Cyclosporine, dihydropyridine calcium channel antagonists (CCAs), phenytoin
Gynecomastia	Antiandrogens, cimetidine, estrogens, griseofulvin, ketoconazole, methyldopa, spironolactone
Hemolysis in glucose-6-phosphate dehydrogenase (G6PD) deficiency	Aspirin, chloramphenicol, dapsone, ibuprofen, isoniazid, nitrofurantoin, primaquine, quinine/quinidine, sulfonamides
Hepatotoxicity	Acetaminophen, cyclophosphamide, erythromycin esto-late, halothane, isoniazid, ketoconazole, lovastatin, niacin, rifampin, valproic acid
Hyperkalemia	Angiotensin-converting enzyme (ACE) inhibitors and angiotensin antagonists, amiloride, cytotoxic drugs, digoxin overdose, heparin, lithium, spironolactone, succinylcholine
Hyperuricemia	Aspirin, cytotoxic drugs, loop and thiazide diuretics, pyrazinamide
Hypokalemia	Corticosteroids, diuretics (osmotics, loop, and thiazides), insulin, sympathomimetics, theophylline
Hyponatremia	Carbamazepine, diuretics, phenothiazines, selective serotonin reuptake inhibitors (SSRIs), venlafaxine, vincristine
Inducers of hepatic cytochrome P-450s	Barbiturates, carbamazepine, ethanol, phenytoin, rifampin, St. John's wort
Inhibitors of hepatic cytochrome P-450s	Cimetidine, erythromycin, ethanol, grapefruit juice, indinavir, ketoconazole, ritonavir
Interstitial nephritis	Ciprofloxacin, furosemide, methicillin, nonsteroidal anti-inflammatory drugs (NSAIDs), sulfonamides

(continued)

Table A–3. Signature drug toxicities. (*Continued*)

Toxicity	Drug or Drug Groups
Phototoxicity	Amiodarone, fluoroquinolones, griseofulvin, pyrazinamide, sulfonamides, tetracyclines, thiazides
Porphyria exacerbation	Barbiturates, estrogens, griseofulvin, oral contraceptives, phenytoin, pyrazinamide, rifampin, sulfonamides
Positive Coombs test	Methyldopa
Pulmonary fibrosis	Amiodarone, bleomycin, busulfan, ergots, procarbazine
Serotonin syndrome with SSRIs	Monoamine oxidase inhibitors (MAOIs), MDMA ("ecstasy"), meperidine, selegiline, tricyclic antidepressants
Systemic lupus erythematosus (SLE)-like syndrome	Hydralazine, isoniazid, methyldopa, procainamide, sulfonamides
Tinnitus	Antimalarials, aspirin, quinidine/quinine

INDEX

Note: Page numbers followed by *t* and *f* indicate tables and figures, respectively.